SHAPE
YOUR
LIFE

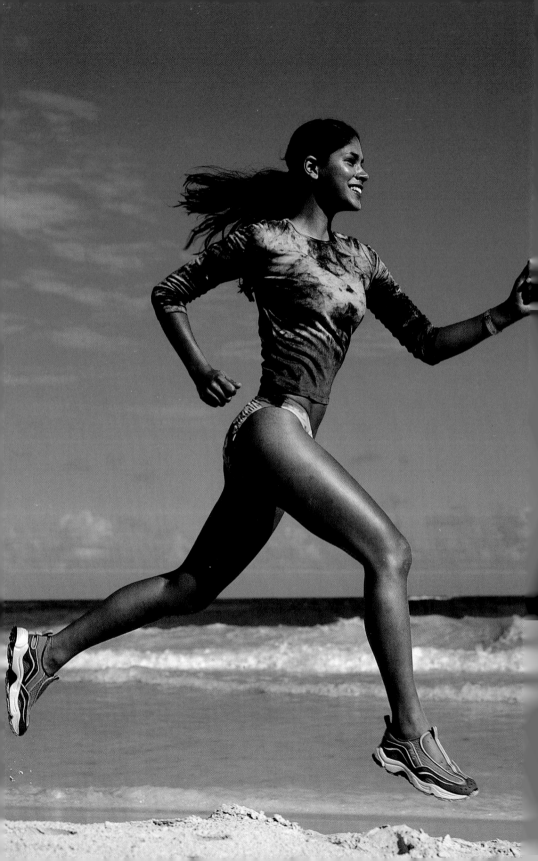

SHAPE
magazine's

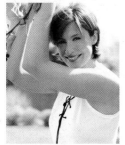

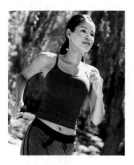

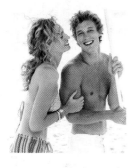

SHAPE YOUR LIFE

4 Weeks to a Better Body—and a Better Life

BARBARA HARRIS,
Editor-in-Chief, *Shape*® magazine,
with Angela Hynes

LIFE
Styles

Hay House, Inc.
Carlsbad, California •
Sydney, Australia •
Canada • Hong Kong •
United Kingdom

PRODUCED BY THE PHILIP LIEF GROUP, INC.

Published and distributed in the United States by: Hay House, Inc., P.O. Box 5100, Carlsbad, CA 92018-5100 • (800) 654-5126 • (800) 650-5115 (fax) • www.hayhouse.com
Published and distributed in Australia by: Hay House Australia Pty Ltd, P.O. Box 515, Brighton-Le-Sands, NSW 2216 • *phone:* 1800 023 516 • *e-mail:* info@hayhouse.com.au
Distributed in the United Kingdom by: Airlift, 8 The Arena, Mollison Ave., Enfield, Middlesex, United Kingdom EN3 7NL • **Distributed in Canada by:** Raincoast, 9050 Shaughnessy St., Vancouver, B.C., Canada V6P 6E5

Editorial supervision: Jill Kramer   *Design:* Summer McStravick

Library of Congress Cataloging-in-Publication Data

Shape your life
    Shape magazine's shape your life : 4 weeks to a better body and a better life / [editors] Barbara Harris, with Angela Hynes.
        p. cm.
    ISBN 1-40190-158-1 (Hardcover) * ISBN 1-4019-0159-X (tradepaper)
    1. Women--Health and hygiene. 2. Physical fitness for women.
    I. Title: Shape your life. II. Harris, Barbara, 1956- III. Hynes, Angela.
IV. Title.
RA778 .S5455 2003
613.7'045--dc21
                            2002013533

Hardcover ISBN 1-4019-0158-1
Tradepaper ISBN 1-4019-0159-X

06 05 04 03   4 3 2 1
1st printing, January 2003

Printed in the United States of America

This book is dedicated to the millions of Shape®

readers in the U.S. and throughout the world.

Your earnest quest for greater well-being has

provided me a continued source of inspiration.

May this information contribute to your

wholeness and joy for life.

— Barbara Harris

contents

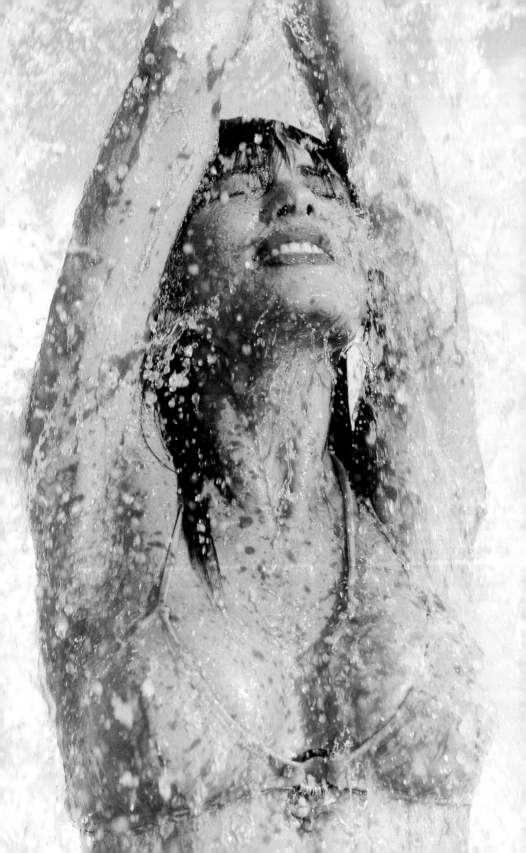

acknowledgments

Thanks are in order to the many people who have made this work possible: Angela Hynes, for her personal commitment to living holistically, her insightful writing, and expedient and tireless efforts in preparing this manuscript; to Anne M. Russell, *Shape*'s editorial director, for her brilliant editing and immediate willingness to take on yet another project; and to Judy Linden and Lynne Kirk at The Philip Lief Group. Their enthusiasm for this book was a gift, and their attention to deadlines facilitated its timely completion. Thanks also to Danny Levin at Hay House, for his immediate love of the *Shape Your Life* concept and his willingness to think outside the box to help spread the message.

Applause is also due others: Fiona Maynard, director of rights and permissions at Weider Publications, for clearing use of content throughout the book; Melissa O'Brien, *Shape*'s director of photography and casting, for her love of *Shape Your Life* and her many hours collaborating with Sally Wilson, art editor at The Philip Lief Group, on carefully choosing the images; Linda Shelton, *Shape*'s fitness editor, for her many years of dedicated work and sharing her uncanny abilities in meticulously translating exercise programs to print; to Robin Vitetta-Miller, for her contribution of recipes for this book; and to the many experts, writers, photographers, and illustrators who have contributed to *Shape*® throughout the years. Their willing contributions, particularly those of *Shape*'s Advisory Board, have enabled the magazine to deliver credible information. The thorough research and talents of many gifted writers and editors have brought the experts' information to life and into the hands of our readers for more than 20 years.

Thanks also to Joe Weider, publisher and founder of *Shape*® magazine; and Christine MacIntyre, founding editor, for their vision and commitment to mind-body fitness and love of the *Shape*® reader; to Eric Weider, president and CEO of Weider Health and Firness; Russell Denson, president and CEO of Weider Publications; and Henry Marks, group publisher, Active Lifestyle (including *Shape*®) at Weider Publications, for their inspiration and support of the magazine and its mission.

The biggest thanks are to the millions of *Shape*® readers—your diligence to getting fit and your trust in the magazine have inspired us and given deep meaning to our daily work; and to our many colleagues, family members, and friends who have inspired us by your friendship, love, patience, and support of our life's work.

Finally, deep gratitude to the handful of experts who have helped translate the *Shape Your Life* concept into living, breathing programs that have love as their foundation. We give thanks for the grace of many blessings, the dedication of many resources, and belief of many in the value of the magazine, this book, and the work that will bloom from the seed of these pages and hopefully give new life to many.

— **Barbara Harris** and the editors of *Shape*® magazine

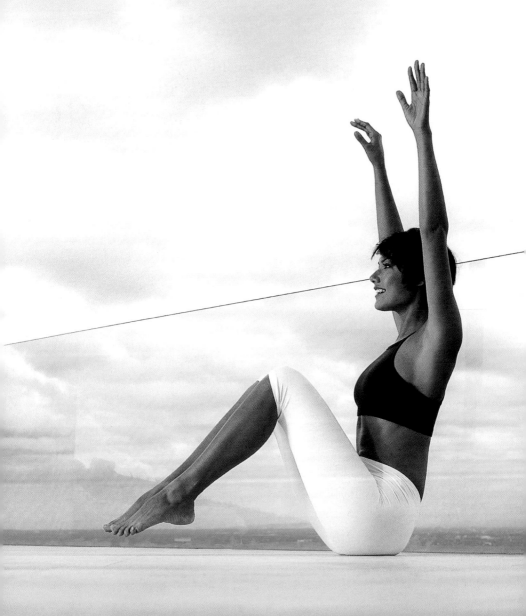

introduction

redefining fitness for a better life

It's time for an entirely new approach to fitness— one that's based upon knowledge of the body's wondrous physiology and compassion for the human spirit.

Regardless of your fitness goal—whether it's to lose weight, to reduce stress, to get your best body ever, or to live your best life—we at *Shape®* do not believe in the "whip yourself into shape" philosophy. The sure and healthy way to get results is to learn to listen to your body and your heart to create a better life.

The punitive, deprivational approach to fitness isn't necessary. Instead of focusing on what you should *not* eat or should *not* do, focus on what foods you *do* need to eat more of to be healthier, what kinds of movement you need to add to feel more alive in your body, and what experiences can help you achieve what you want in life.

Even if your sole aim is to get flatter abs or a firmer butt, your surest route to success is to go beyond improving your exercise and diet regimens alone. Achieving your best physical results requires that you expand your focus to encompass shaping your entire life. To that end, *Shape®* has identified seven elements that are essential for total fitness: *exercise, a healthy diet, spirituality* (to nurture your inner self), *adequate rest* (including sleep and relaxation), *emotional well-being, a healthy body image* (which promotes a positive view of and a new relationship with your body at any size or shape), and *work* that is both satisfying and rewarding.

Fitness is a web of relationships among these seven elements. Each impacts the others, and each has the power to contribute significantly to your health and well-being. For example, unhappiness at work can sap your energy (leaving you too tired to exercise), and can eventually erode your health; it can even leave you too drained to be a good partner in your relationship. Research also shows that inadequate sleep may lead you to overeat and manage stressful situations poorly. On the other hand, getting the rest you need boosts immunity and enhances learning and creativity. Likewise, exercise not only reduces your risk for heart disease, cancer, and diabetes, but it also can effectively treat depression and reduce work stress (even a two-minute walk can lessen anxiety). And the list goes on: Having supportive primary relationships boosts immunity; living in an environment that nurtures your healthy lifestyle may help you adhere to healthy living practices for the long term; and nourishing and exercising your spiritual beliefs may have profound positive effects on your total well-being.

Body image, in particular, is an element of fitness that's been long underrated and misunderstood. So many women feel that they'd be happier if they were just a smaller size or more toned. Although feeling "good" about our bodies is often related to having high self-esteem, feeling "bad" about something in our lives often gets projected onto our bodies when we suddenly "feel fat." According to a recent survey of 7,000 *Shape*® magazine readers, we don't feel good about ourselves when we overeat either. The primary reasons for overeating are being bored, stressed, depressed, or lonely. If you eat to soothe your emotions, you may have found that you can't stop overeating simply by saying that you're not going to do it anymore. We need to learn the techniques for managing our emotions.

We can learn to tune in to our bodies and our hearts and nourish them in ways that are good for us. Hundreds of studies spanning decades of research in mind-body fitness, health, psychology, and medicine provide overwhelming evidence for a holistic approach to fitness for optimum health and well-being. That's what *Shape Your Life* is all about. Regardless of where you are in your quest for fitness, health, and happiness, you can further your progress. In this book, chapter by chapter, you'll learn how to master each of the seven elements of fitness by using the easy-to-apply four-week programs, quick tips, and mistakes to avoid. For example, you'll learn how to do the following:

- Test your overall fitness; boost your aerobic capacity, strength, and flexibility; achieve a healthy weight; and feel body confident **(Chapter 1: Your Workout)**.

- Create an eating plan that fits your lifestyle based on adding satisfying and delicious foods to your diet, including what you need to eat more of to be leaner and healthier **(Chapter 2: Your Diet)**.

- Improve your spiritual fitness, whether through exploring new connections, religious practices or belief systems, journaling, or simply spending more time in nature **(Chapter 3: Your Spirituality)**.

- Develop a renewed appreciation for sleep, rest, and relaxation; learn how to enhance the quality of your sleep; and make every vacation restorative. In fact, sleep may be the one missing link in your fitness program **(Chapter 4: Your Rest)**.

- Become more optimistic, establish richer relationships, kick bad habits, and soothe stress. We want you to do more than survive—we want you to find joy **(Chapter 5: Your Emotions)**!

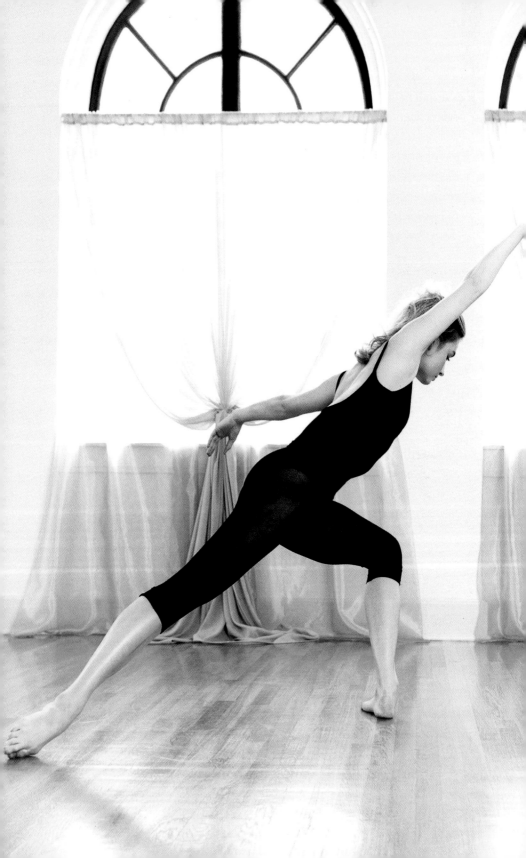

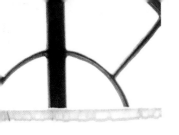

- Get "Body Confident," discover how to counter "emotional eating," and formulate realistic goals. You'll develop a new relationship with your body and a new view of it **(Chapter 6: Your Body Image)**.

- Make work satisfying and rewarding, learn to banish burnout, and stay healthy on the job—whether you're self-employed, have a job in a large corporation, or are fully employed as a homemaker and mother. You'll even be able to figure out if you have a bad job—or just an attitude that needs adjusting **(Chapter 7: Work)**.

Robert Ivker, D.O., and past president of the American Holistic Medical Association, says that a powerful predictor of your health is your answer to these two questions: "Do you love your life?" and "Are you happy to be alive?" Recognize the futility of having flat abs if your life is mediocre or bereft of meaning. Make the goals of your fitness program to feel alive in your body and to simply live your best life. *Shape Your Life* provides the tools to help you do that. The result: You'll not only get your best body ever, but you'll also enjoy your best health and your most incredible life.

My best to you,
— **Barbara Harris,** Editor-in-Chief, *Shape*® magazine

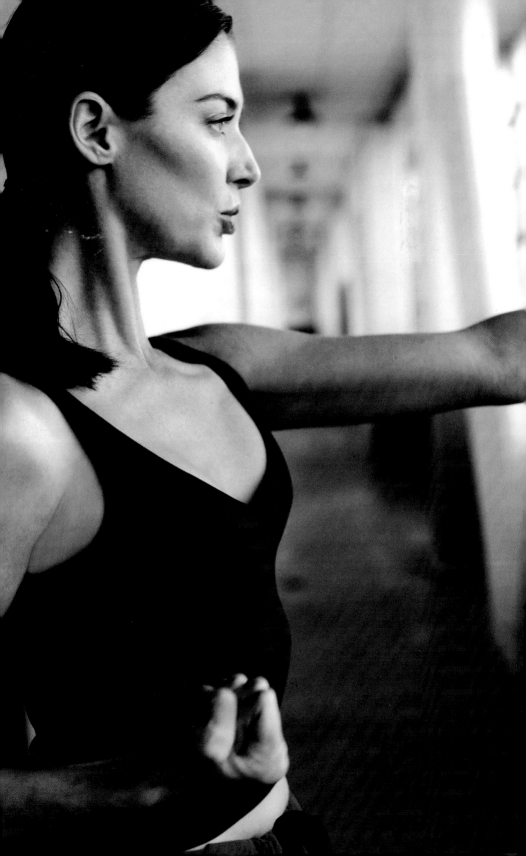

your workout

Quick Tip: *Make every exercise session mindful by quieting mental chatter and shifting focus inward to your body's working muscles and rhythmic breathing.*

what you'll learn

Shape's approach to working out is that physical activity is a cornerstone of total wellness. We'll help you formulate an exercise plan that incorporates exercise into your daily life based on your health status, lifestyle, and fitness goals. Using this chapter, you'll:

- boost your energy with aerobic activity
- sculpt your muscles by strength training
- work out even when you think you have no time
- exercise mindfully
- become flexible by stretching
- achieve and maintain a healthy weight
- become body confident

how you'll do it

Over the years, we've learned at *Shape®* that there's much more to fitness than meets the eye. Sure, most of us want tight abs, lean legs, and toned triceps—but we also exercise to be healthy, feel comfortable in our skin, and have energy for activities other than work.

In terms of health, study after study has confirmed that staying active on a regular, long-term basis—and it's only too late if you never start—can help prevent or delay diseases such as colon and breast cancer, high blood pressure, heart disease, stroke, osteoporosis, and diabetes. Exercise also helps to elevate "good" (HDL) cholesterol, boosts your

> **Quick Tip:** *Hire a short-term trainer who can offer custom-tailored solutions for you. In just one or two sessions, a trainer can help identify poor technique and other reasons your workouts aren't as effective as they could be.*

immune system to reduce your incidence of colds and flu, and promotes healthy muscles and joints. There's nothing quite as efficient as an active lifestyle for keeping you looking and feeling younger longer. Recent research also suggests that exercise helps prevent the loss of mental reasoning and creativity as you age.

These are all long-term benefits, but if you're more likely to be motivated by short-term, if not instant, gratification, consider this: Exercise can blast off fat; improve your mood; relieve stress; give your sex life a lift; enhance work, recreation, and sports performance; help you kick bad habits; improve the quality of your sleep; and make your skin glow. For women facing menopause, exercise may relieve some of the symptoms that may accompany its onset, such as mood swings and insomnia. And as you become increasingly fit, you'll probably gain body confidence and boost self-esteem.

Just as you must eat a variety of foods for proper nutrition, you need several types of exercise to maintain and improve fitness—cardio, stretching, and strength training. How much do you need of each? Here's a realistic and healthy guideline for all three types:

cardio exercise

Duration: For health, almost daily for 30 minutes total of moderate activity (research suggests three 10-minute sessions may be just as good as one 30-minute session). For fitness, moderate to vigorous aerobic exercise 3–5 days a week for 20–60 minutes. For weight loss and maintenance, you may need up to one hour of regular, moderate activity, such as continuous walking at a brisk pace.

Rationale: Reduces your risk for heart disease, diabetes, high blood pressure, colon cancer, and many other conditions. Weight-bearing exercises such as running and walking also help prevent osteoporosis.

stretching

Duration: Almost daily for 5–10 minutes. Stretch each major muscle group (see "The Sexy Side of Stretching," page 43), holding each stretch to a point of mild tension for 10–30 seconds without bouncing.

Rationale: Keeps you flexible and your joints mobile, may reduce your risk of injury and improve your quality of life.

total body strength training

Duration: Twice a week, at least one set of 8–12 repetitions using enough weight to fatigue each muscle group.

Rationale: May strengthen your bones; keeps your muscles strong and your metabolism humming.

fitness test

Before you start a new workout regimen, it's a good idea to assess your current level of cardio fitness and strength. (If you're embarking on an exercise program for the very first time, you may want to consult with your doctor before starting.) Take our fitness test and record how you did and how you felt on our scorecard on the next page. You'll discover where your weaknesses lie, and which of our workouts best suits your needs. Retake the tests at the end of the month. You should see a noticeable improvement in your scores, and feel more energized and confident about your abilities as you progress.

strength

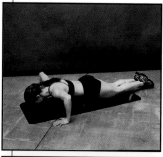

1. Upper-Body Test. Do as many bent-knee push-ups as you can with good form (no time limit).

Kneel with hands just ahead of shoulders, arms straight, and body forming one straight line from head to hips. Bend elbows to lower body until they're even with your shoulders and chest is about three inches from floor (shown), then straighten arms to push back up to the starting position.

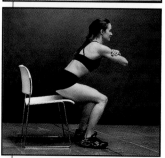

2. Lower-Body Test. Do as many chair squats as you can with good form (no time limit).

Stand in front of a sturdy chair, feet hip-width apart. Cross arms over chest. Keeping body weight over heels, lower torso (shown) until the back of your thighs touch the chair seat. Take four seconds to lower and two seconds to stand.

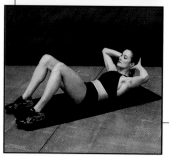

3. Abdominal Test. Do as many crunches as you can in one minute, using good form.

Lie face up with knees bent and feet flat on the floor. Place hands behind head, fingers touching but not clasped. Curl head, neck, and shoulders up until shoulder blades clear the floor (shown), then lower shoulders to floor.

cardio

The Cooper Institute's Aerobic Fitness Test. Time yourself as you run, jog, or walk for one and a half miles on flat terrain (outdoors or on a treadmill). If you can't run the whole way, start off walking and gradually pick up the pace. Do your best, but don't overexert yourself. Before and after the test, be sure to walk for several minutes to let your body warm up and cool down. Wait at least two hours after eating to take this test.

YOUR SCORECARD

Upper Body

20 Number of push-ups

How I felt afterward *tired, disappointed*

Lower Body

25 Number of chair squats

How I felt afterward *fine — could have kept going*

Abdominals

50 Number of crunches

How I felt afterward *could have kept going*

Cardio

15:25 Time

How I felt afterward *VERY disappointed - out of shape!*

what the numbers mean

Note: This data provides a range of scores for the average woman. Roughly speaking, women ages 20–29 should be looking at the higher end of the range, women 30–39 at the mid range, and women over 40 at the lower end of the range.

	Upper-Body Strength (push-ups)	Lower-Body Strength (chair squats)	Abdominal Strength (crunches)	Walk/Run Time (cardio)
Excellent	33 or more	25 or more	48 or more	Below 12:50
Good	22–32	20–24	37–47	12:51–14:23
Average	10–21	15–19	25–36	*
Fair	0–9	10–14	13–24	14:24–15:25
Poor	0	0–9	0–13	Above 15:26

*The Cooper Institute does not use this rating in its Aerobic Fitness Test.

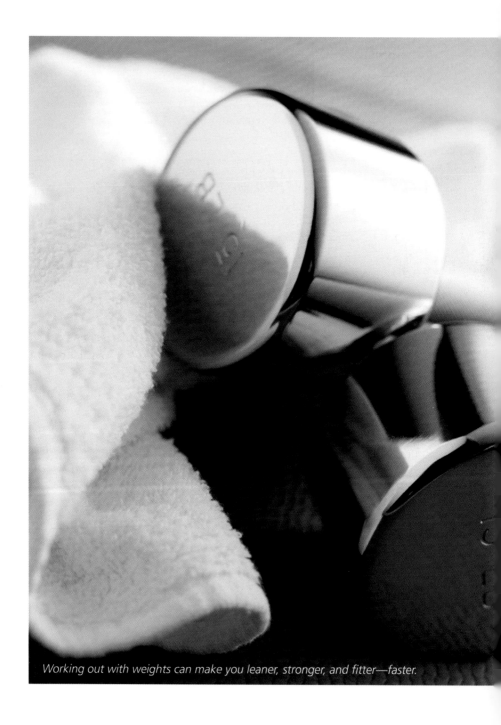

Working out with weights can make you leaner, stronger, and fitter—faster.

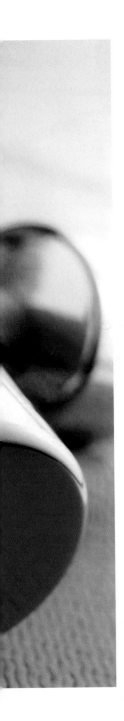

Since we all have varying fitness goals and lifestyles, there's no single workout routine that's right for everyone. While some get their cardio workouts from running outdoors, others prefer a stair climber at the gym or jumping rope on their balcony. Many women need the group energy that's generated by a class, while others prefer the meditative quality of working out alone.

Just as there are myriad ways to work out, there are just as many motivations for doing so. And researchers have discovered that what motivates you best determines whether you'll keep exercising. If you'd rather take a pill than exercise or improve your diet, your motivation to exercise is probably external: to look good or to lose weight. But if you derive pleasure from engaging in exercise and how it makes you feel, you're internally driven, and there's a higher likelihood that you'll stick with it. With your own motivation in mind, select one or more of the four *Shape Your Life* workouts that's right for you.

the ultra-efficient walk-run cardio workout

It used to be that there were women who walked and women who ran. Not anymore. Today's runners often take walking breaks to give their joints a rest, while walkers add jogging to their workout for increased intensity.

"Choosing whether to run or walk is really a matter of personal taste," says Therese Iknoian, the author of *Walking Fast* and *Fitness Walking,* who designed this four-week program. "If you like the feeling of springing through the air and lengthening your stride, you'll want to build into a run. But if the impact doesn't feel good to you, walking briskly is an equally demanding workout."

As well as having considerable health benefits, walk-run cardio workouts can burn significant calories while sending your spirits soaring. Melissa Hicks, a *Shape®* reader from Long Beach, California, does her cardio workout on the beach. "The crisp ocean air and the sound of the waves and seagulls always improve my mood, and walking and running on the sand boosts my heart rate," she says.

Although you can get cardio exercise on gym equipment such as stair climbers or rowing machines, the beauty of this workout is that all you really need is a good pair of shoes and somewhere to walk . . . or run . . . or both.

Although you can burn about the same number of calories, mile for mile, whether you're walking or running, there's one important difference between the two activities: time. If you take 28–30 minutes to cover three miles running, you may need about 45 minutes to cover those same three miles at a brisk walk. So, it takes longer to burn the same amount of calories walking as it does running.

Here's a specific example: A 145-pound woman walking three miles per hour burns 145 calories in 30 minutes, while the same woman burns 393 calories running at about seven miles per hour for the same amount of time. The trade-off is that running takes more of a toll on your body because of its high-impact nature.

Our walk-run program makes the best of both worlds. You'll save time but still have a chance to enjoy your surroundings and burn lots of calories. The intervals will make each workout interesting and fun. No matter what your fitness level is, this program will build your cardio endurance and leave you feeling great.

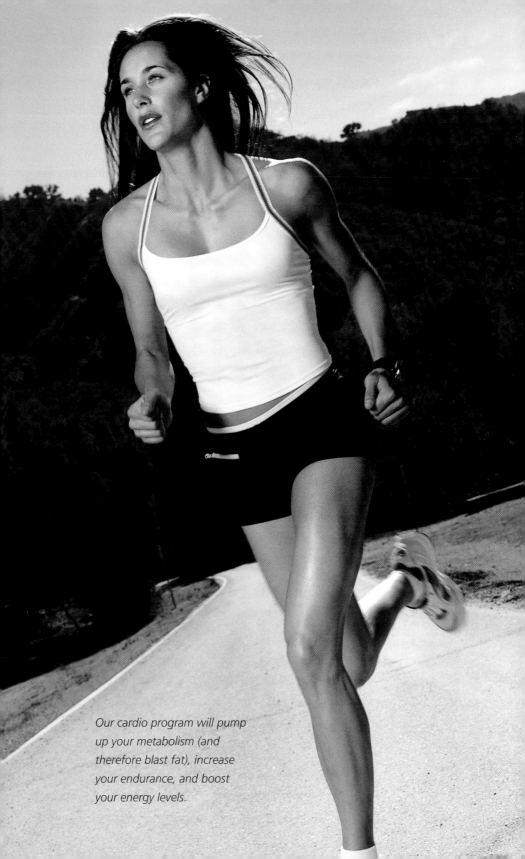

Our cardio program will pump up your metabolism (and therefore blast fat), increase your endurance, and boost your energy levels.

how hard are you working?

For aerobic exercise to be effective, you should exercise in your target heart rate zone. But what is that? The standard formula is to subtract your age from 220, then work within 60 to 90 percent of that figure. There's a simpler way to judge your heart rate that's relatively accurate—use the rate of perceived exertion (RPE) scale to estimate the intensity of your workout session. Here's how it breaks down:

RPE Intensity Level

1–2   Very easy; you can converse with no effort.
3   Easy; you can converse with almost no effort.
4   Moderately easy; you can converse comfortably with little effort.
5   Moderate; conversation requires some effort.
6   Moderately hard; conversation requires quite a bit of effort.
7   Difficult; conversation requires a lot of effort.
8   Very difficult; conversation requires maximum effort
9–10 Peak exertion; no-talking zone.

the plan

Each workout in this four-week program incorporates running into a walking workout using interval walk-run sets. For each interval, run for a number of minutes (say, 3 or 4) and then walk for the same number. Then repeat. "Walk-runners should not move from a stroll to a sprint," says walking expert Therese Iknoian. "The running part of the interval should only be a tad more intense than a very brisk walk."

For example, if you were using an effort scale that goes from 1 (not moving at all) to 10 (working at a peak level), the walks would be at a level 4, 5, or 6; while the runs would be at a level 5, 6, or 7.

Before moving to the next week, you should be comfortably accomplishing the current week's workout. If not, repeat that week's workouts as many sessions as needed before moving on. If the workouts described are too short or too long, simply add or subtract a set of run-walk intervals, as needed.

The workout progresses from longer walks to long runs, but if you prefer walking to running, feel free to stick with the week's worth of programs that you enjoy the most; however, see if you can increase your intensity.

week one: three alternating days

Monday: *31 minutes*

- Warm up by walking slowly for 5 minutes.
- Stretch out leg muscles gently for 2 minutes.
- Walk for 8 minutes at a steady pace.
- Do two "walk-run" sets: Alternate 1 minute of fast walking with 3 minutes of moderate speed walking.
- Cool down by reducing your pace for 3 minutes until you reach a comfortable walking pace.
- Full-body stretch for 5 minutes (see "The Sexy Side of Stretching," page 43).

Wednesday: *45 minutes*

- Warm up by walking slowly for 5 minutes.
- Stretch out leg muscles gently for 2 minutes.
- Walk at a moderate pace for 15 minutes. Then begin 3 run-walk sets: Alternate running for 1 minute with walking for 4 minutes.
- Cool down by reducing your pace for 3 minutes until you reach a comfortable walking pace.
- Full-body stretch for 5 minutes.

Friday: *43 minutes*

- Warm up by walking slowly for 5 minutes.
- Stretch out leg muscles gently for 2 minutes.
- Walk at a moderate pace for 12 minutes. Then begin 4 run-walk sets: Alternate running for 1 minute with walking for 3 minutes.
- Cool down by reducing your pace for 3 minutes until you reach a comfortable walking pace.
- Full-body stretch for 5 minutes.

week two: four alternating days

Monday: *35–40 minutes*

1/19

- Warm up by walking slowly for 5 minutes.
- Stretch out leg muscles gently for 2 minutes.
- Walk briskly for 8–10 minutes. Then begin 3–4 speed-play sets: Alternate fast walking for 1 minute with moderate speed walking for 3 minutes.
- Cool down by reducing your pace for 3 minutes until you reach a comfortable walking pace.
- Full-body stretch for 5 minutes.

Tuesday: *50 minutes*

11/20

- Warm up by walking slowly for 5 minutes.
- Stretch out leg muscles gently for 2 minutes.
- Walk at a moderate pace for 12 minutes. Then begin 3 run-walk sets: Alternate running for 2 minutes with walking for 3 minutes. Finally, run for 2 minutes, walk for 6 minutes.
- Cool down by reducing your pace for 3 minutes until you reach a comfortable walking pace.
- Full-body stretch for 5 minutes.

Thursday: *43 minutes*

11/22

- Warm up by walking slowly for 5 minutes.
- Stretch out leg muscles gently for 2 minutes.
- Walk at a moderate pace for 8 minutes. Then begin 5 speed-play sets: Alternate fast walking for 1 minute with moderate speed walking for 3 minutes.
- Cool down by reducing your pace for 3 minutes until you reach a comfortable walking pace.
- Full-body stretch for 5 minutes.

Saturday: *45 minutes*

11/24

- Warm up by walking slowly for 5 minutes.
- Stretch out leg muscles gently for 2 minutes.
- Walk 10 minutes. Then begin 5 run-walk sets: Alternate running for 2 minutes with walking for 2 minutes.
- Cool down by reducing your pace for 3 minutes until you reach a comfortable walking pace.
- Full-body stretch for 5 minutes.

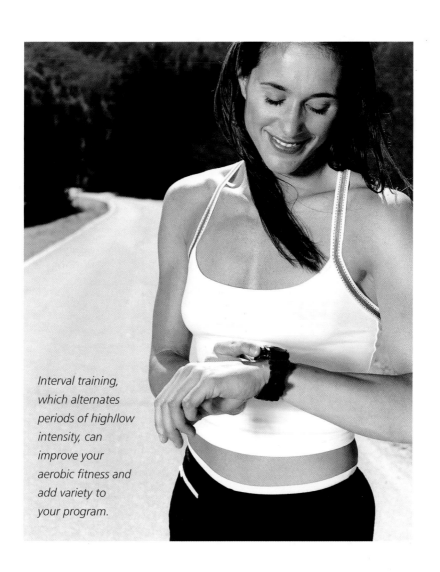

Interval training, which alternates periods of high/low intensity, can improve your aerobic fitness and add variety to your program.

week three: four alternating days
(optional fifth day)

Monday: *43 minutes*

1/27

- Warm up by walking slowly for 5 minutes.
- Stretch out leg muscles gently for 2 minutes.
- Walk at a moderate pace for 8 minutes. Then begin 5 run-walk sets: Alternate running for 2 minutes with walking for 2 minutes.
- Cool down by reducing your pace for 3 minutes until you reach a comfortable walking pace.
- Full-body stretch for 5 minutes.

Wednesday: *48 minutes*

1/28

- Warm up by walking slowly for 5 minutes.
- Stretch out leg muscles gently for 2 minutes.
- Walk 6 minutes. Then begin 4 run-walk sets: Alternate running for 3 minutes with walking for 2 minutes. Finally, run for 3 minutes, walk for 4 minutes.
- Cool down by reducing your pace for 3 minutes until you reach a comfortable walking pace.
- Full-body stretch for 5 minutes.

Thursday: *55 minutes*

- Warm up by walking slowly for 5 minutes.
- Stretch out leg muscles gently for 2 minutes.
- Walk 10 minutes. Then begin 6 run-walk sets: Alternate running for 2 minutes with walking for 2 minutes. Finally, run 2 minutes, walk 4 minutes.
- Cool down by reducing your pace for 3 minutes until you reach a comfortable walking pace.
- Full-body stretch for 5 minutes.

Saturday: *55 minutes*

- Warm up by walking slowly for 5 minutes.
- Stretch out leg muscles gently for 2 minutes.
- Walk 4 minutes. Then begin 5 run-walk sets: Alternate running for 4 minutes with walking for 2 minutes. Finally, run 2 minutes, walk 4 minutes.
- Cool down by reducing your pace for 3 minutes until you reach a comfortable walking pace.
- Full-body stretch for 5 minutes.

Optional Fifth Day: *30-minute walk*

week four: four alternating days
(optional fifth day)

Monday: *49 minutes*
- Warm up by walking slowly for 5 minutes.
- Stretch out leg muscles gently for 2 minutes.
- Walk 4 minutes. Then begin 5 run-walk sets: Alternate running for 4 minutes with walking for 1 minute. Finally, run 1 minute, walk 4 minutes.
- Cool down by reducing your pace for 3 minutes until you reach a comfortable walking pace.
- Full-body stretch for 5 minutes.

Wednesday: *47 minutes*
- Warm up by walking slowly for 5 minutes.
- Stretch out leg muscles gently for 2 minutes.
- Walk 2 minutes. Then begin 4 run-walk sets: Alternate running for 5 minutes with walking for 1 minute. Finally, run 2 minutes, walk 4 minutes.
- Cool down by reducing your pace for 3 minutes until you reach a comfortable walking pace.
- Full-body stretch for 5 minutes.

Thursday: *51 minutes*
- Warm up by walking slowly for 5 minutes.
- Stretch out leg muscles gently for 2 minutes.
- Walk 8 minutes. Then begin 6 run-walk sets: Alternate running for 2 minutes with walking for 2 minutes. Finally, run 2 minutes, walk 2 minutes.
- Cool down by reducing your pace for 3 minutes until you reach a comfortable walking pace.
- Full-body stretch for 5 minutes.

Saturday: *50 minutes*
- Warm up by walking slowly for 5 minutes.
- Stretch out leg muscles gently for 2 minutes.
- Walk 1 minute. Then begin 3 run-walk sets: Alternate running for 8 minutes with walking for 1 minute. Finally, walk 6 minutes, run 1 minute.
- Cool down by reducing your pace for 3 minutes until you reach a comfortable walking pace.
- Full-body stretch for 5 minutes.

Optional Fifth Day: *Repeat Monday's workout*

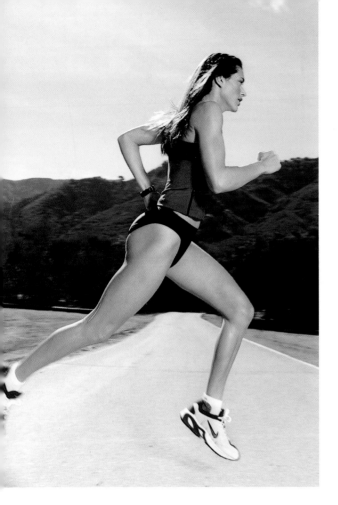

Form: Form is similar for running and walking. Strive for a natural stride, and keep your torso erect. Always stabilize body position with your abdominal muscles. Keep shoulders and hands relaxed (but don't round shoulders), bend elbows at about 90 degrees, and drive forearms forward and back like the piston rods on a steam locomotive (avoid pumping them up and down, which wastes momentum and energy). Keep your chin parallel to the ground, and look straight ahead. Let your foot roll heel-to-toe through its full range of motion—don't slap it down.

Walking Only: To make your walking as intense as running, focus on technique, which will help you go faster. Move your feet quickly, and drive arms to match their speed. Don't try to achieve speed by taking longer strides, which is potentially harmful to your back. Try hiking hills for a real jolt. Forget hand and ankle weights—they don't do much to increase intensity and may cause injury.

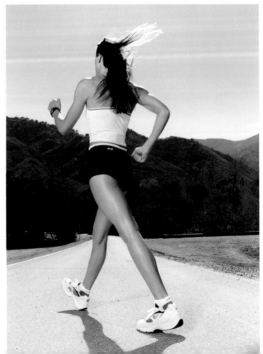

picking up the aerobic pace

As you become more fit, the workouts that used to invigorate you instead leave you stuck in a rut. You run those same three miles at a plodding pace. Or you faithfully show up for step aerobics but can't seem to lose any more fat. When that happens, you need to kick up the intensity of your aerobic workout. Here are some expert tips to help you boost your calorie burn and improve your endurance:

- Add intervals to your cardio workouts. For 1–2 workouts per week, alternate 30–60 seconds of high-intensity exercise with three times as much slower-paced exercise (also called "active rest"), then repeat the interval 5–10 more times. As you become more fit, increase the length of your high-intensity exercise and decrease the length of the slower paced activity, eventually aiming for a 1:1 hard/easy radio. For every 1-mph increase in your pace, you'll burn about 25 percent more calories. Translation: Walking at 4.5 mph, a 145-pound woman will burn 425 calories in an hour, compared to 309 calories at 3 mph.

- Add hills to your workouts. For every 2 percent grade increase, you'll burn approximately 25 percent more calories walking. Plus, you'll boost your fitness level. Try hill "repeats" once a week: Find a hill that you can climb in 3–5 minutes at about 80 percent of your maximum heart rate. Start with 2 or 3 repeats, and gradually work up to five.

- Train for an event, such as a 10K run or a mini-triathlon. The moment you mail your entry fee, you'll have a new sense of purpose and a concrete goal that will push you to achieve more.

- Join a club or team. Become a member of a bicycling club, a walking group, a swimming team, a soccer league, or another activity-related organization in your area. Working with a group always encourages competition, which pushes you to higher levels.

the fit-in-20-minutes workout

One of the most common reasons people give for not working out is lack of time. But that's not really a legitimate excuse, and we can prove it!

You don't have to spend hours in the gym to maintain your definition. For those of you who plead "time crunch," we've come up with a workout that will strengthen and tone your whole body in just 20 minutes the first couple of weeks, and in 30 when you work up to the maximum number of sets. Let's face it, even the busiest of us can carve out 30 minutes from our day: How about watching one less TV sitcom?

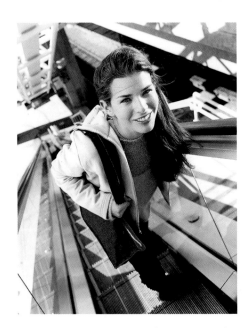

Always rushing? You don't have to spend hours in the gym to maintain your fitness.

We asked Juan Carlos Santana, M.Ed., C.S.C.S., director of Optimum Performance Systems in Boca Raton, Florida, to design a dumbbell routine that's the fastest total-body workout you can do. He picked five moves, two of which are challenging twists on familiar exercises—namely, one-arm rows and push-ups. The others are compound exercises consisting of two or three strength moves that hit multiple muscle groups all at once.

"With these kinds of compound moves, you're doing several back-to-back exercises as one exercise without resting between sets, which helps you save time," Santana says. You also burn more calories because you're working your muscles and your heart harder.

Dumbbells can be more time-efficient and effective than weight machines. Free-standing exercises require using your ab and low-back muscles to stabilize your body, so you get a bonus "core" workout.

You'll need a set of 5– to 15–pound dumbbells to start. For each move, select a weight that feels challenging but allows you to complete all reps with good form. With compound exercises, you work more than one muscle group at once, so you may need to use a lighter weight than usual in order to complete all portions of the exercise. In other words, you normally might do squats with two 15-pound dumbbells, but for biceps curls, you can only lift 10 pounds. So, you would want to use 10-pound weights for the squat, curl, and press. The bottom line is, you're only as strong as your weakest muscle.

Mistake to Avoid: *Don't hit the tennis court, ski slopes, soccer field, or basketball court without preparing with a comprehensive program that includes strength, flexibility, balance, and agility training. Taking up a sport is a great way to be physically active, but you need to be fit enough to avoid injury.*

the plan

Do these moves 2–3 times a week on alternating days. For each move, aim to do 2–4 sets of 8–12 reps, resting 45 seconds between sets. For moves focusing on only one side of the body (#2 and #4), one rep isn't completed until you've done the full exercise on both sides. If this workout doesn't fatigue your muscles, increase your reps to 15 per set or use heavier dumbbells. Based on 2 sets, use the first week to adjust your weight and reps so you're challenged, but can complete the recommended reps with as much weight as you can handle. The second week, increase your weight by 2–3 pounds, decreasing reps if necessary. The third week, increase weight, or, if that's too difficult, keep the weight the same and increase reps by 2–3 for each exercise. The fourth week, do exercises 1 through 6 as a superset or circuit (one exercise right after the other before resting for 1–2 minutes), then repeat for desired sets. After four weeks, go back to lifting 2–4 sets and recommended reps for each exercise, increasing your weight by 10 percent.

Start each workout with a two- to three-minute warm-up: Walk briskly, do jumping jacks, do alternating knee lifts, use the cardio machine of your choice—or do the moves in the workout without weights. After each workout, do static stretches for all your major muscles groups (see "The Sexy Side of Stretching," page 43).

As you get stronger, add resistance (go up in dumbbell weight) so that your muscles stay challenged. To avoid plateaus, change exercises and progress in intensity. You can do so by splitting compound exercises into single moves (for example, break down the squat, curl, and press by doing all of your squats, followed by all of your biceps curls, and then all of your overhead presses).

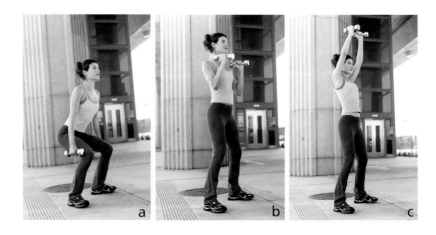

1. Squat, curl, and press. *Holding dumbbells, stand with feet hip-width apart, legs straight, arms hanging by your sides, palms facing in. Contract abdominals so your pelvis is in a neutral position. With body weight toward your heels, bend knees into a squat, lowering torso until thighs are close to parallel to the floor (a). Straighten legs; keeping elbows lined up under shoulders, bend elbows into a curl, raising dumbbells toward shoulders (b). Straighten arms, pressing weight overhead, rotating arms so palms face in, keeping shoulders down and shoulder blades together (c). Lower to starting position.*

Strengthens buttocks, hamstrings, quadriceps, biceps, shoulders, and upper back.

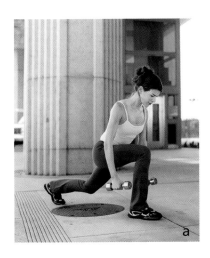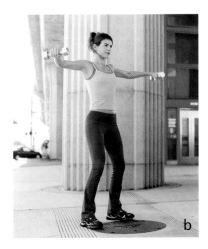

2. Alternating reaching lunge and lateral raise. *Standing in the same starting position as move #1, take a big step forward with your right foot, bending your right knee into a lunge; right knee should be in line with your right ankle, left knee bent and heel lifted. Bend forward from your hips, reaching both arms forward so dumbbells are on either side of your right foot (a). Straighten torso, return dumbbells to sides, then press off your back foot and straighten legs back to starting position. After your body is erect, do a lateral raise, lifting arms out to your sides to shoulder height; keep elbows slightly bent and even with your wrists (b). Lower arms to starting position and repeat entire move, this time stepping forward with your left foot.*

Strengthens quadriceps, hamstrings, buttocks, calves, and middle shoulders; works back and abdominal muscles as stabilizers.

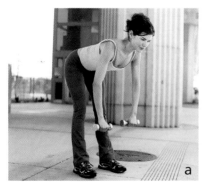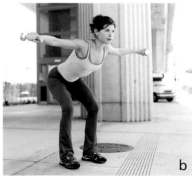

3. Dead lift and bent-over fly. *Stand, feet hip-width apart, legs straight (not locked), holding dumbbells in front of thighs, palms facing you. Contract abdominals and squeeze shoulder blades together. Keeping spine neutral, do a dead lift, bending forward from your hips just until you feel your hamstrings begin to stretch (a). Then, bend knees slightly, squeeze shoulder blades together, and lift arms out to your sides, elbows slightly bent, into a rear fly (b), then lower weights to thighs. Contract your buttocks and return to starting position.*

Strengthens hamstrings, buttocks, rear shoulders, and upper back.

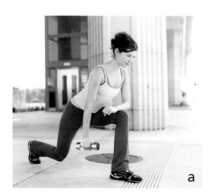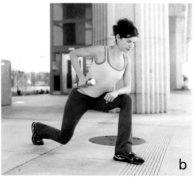

4. Free-standing one-arm row. *Holding a dumbbell in your right hand, stand, feet hip-width apart with your left foot about 2 feet in front of your right. Bend your left leg and place left forearm on left thigh; lean forward from your hips until your upper body is at 45 degrees to the floor (if needed, hold on to a chair). Let right arm hang in line with right shoulder, palm facing in. Contract abs to align head, neck, spine, and hips (a). Squeeze shoulder blades together; then contracting back muscles, bend right elbow up and back toward your waist (b). Straighten arm and repeat with left arm for all reps.*

Strengthens middle back, rear shoulder, and some biceps.

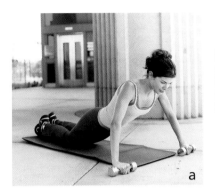
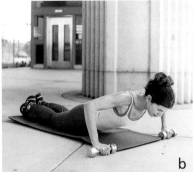

5. Dumbbell push-ups. *Kneel on a mat, holding dumbbells on the floor wider then shoulder-width apart, palms facing floor. Extend a leg at a time behind you until you're supported on your toes, your body in a straight line from head to heels: if needed, rest knees on floor (a). Lower torso by bending arms until forearms and upper arms form 90-degree angles (b). Push up to starting position.*

Strengthens chest, front shoulder, and triceps.

10 ways to keep fitness from fizzling

1. *Know your mission.* Write down why you're trying to get in shape and how will it improve your life. Then read it over when you're tempted to skip a workout.

2. *Dangle a few carrots.* At the end of each week or month that you've stuck to your program, reward your successes with a healthy treat: perhaps a massage or new running shoes.

3. *Plan.* Schedule your workout sessions and write them down on your calendar. Treat them as important appointments that can't be missed.

4. *Track your progress.* A workout journal can help you stay focused on your goals. For each sweat session, record the date, duration, what you did, and how you felt afterward.

5. *Do something active every day.* Even if you can't fit in your full scheduled workout, do a scaled-back one. It's easier to stay on the wagon than to get back on when you've fallen off.

6. *Be a problem solver.* Don't let temporary setbacks like a time crunch or injury derail you. Switch your schedule around or try a new activity.

7. *Think like a pro.* Athletes don't wonder *if* but *when* they'll go to the gym. Establish healthy boundaries to stop other activities from encroaching on your workout times.

8. *Find a reliable training partner.* When you're meeting a friend, it's harder to blow off your workout. Plus, the camaraderie and competition make it more fun.

9. *Believe that change is possible.* Stop thinking that you're destined to be out-of-shape. People who succeed believe that they have control and can make it happen.

10. *Have fun.* You have to like it if you're going to stick with it! Try different workouts until you find the one that floats your boat. Boredom is the ultimate motivation killer.

the body-confident workout

When it comes to building a better body image, not all workouts are created equal. While a variety of physical activities may help you feel better about the way you look, many people believe that pumping iron is an especially effective way to boost your body confidence. Sonnie Thomas, a *Shape®* reader from Des Moines, Iowa, says that joining a gym was "the best thing I could have done. I've reshaped my body and gained so much confidence that I walk proudly with my shoulders back, abs tight, and a big smile. I feel comfortable in my own skin because I've worked hard for it."

Unless you're a real beginner, we're not talking about using dainty three-pound dumbbells or doing a basic circuit of weight machines. Heavier weights and new exercises are the keys to increasing strength and body confidence. We asked former competitive power lifter Jan Todd, Ph.D., assistant professor of kinesiology at the University of Texas at Austin, to design a program to help you build overall body strength and make you feel strong and powerful.

Part of Todd's strategy includes using free weights (dumbbells and barbells) instead of machines. "Many machines are built so that the weight is hidden within a stack, so you don't get a visual sense of how much you're lifting," she says. "With free-weight training, you can see how much you're lifting, which is a helpful visual cue." Free weights also provide a better workout because more muscles are involved.

Mistake to Avoid: *Don't be afraid of using heavy weights. Many women worry that weights will make them bulk up. But that fear is groundless, since we simply don't have enough testosterone to build bulging muscles.*

If you're thinking about pumping iron, you might need to get over any fear or misconceptions you have about what lifting heavy weights will do to your body: You'll get leaner, not bigger. Todd says to find a training partner who can "spot" you so you have the courage to try new moves or lift more weight.

the plan

This four-week program is based on the theory of progressive resistance: In other words, you'll make small increases in the amount of weight you lift and reduce the number of reps each week. Week one you'll do 10 reps per set; weeks two and three you'll do 8 reps per set; and week four you'll do 6 reps per set. To develop strength and muscle tone, lift a weight heavy enough so that the last 2 reps of every set are a struggle, but not so challenging that your form gets sloppy. Depending on how strong you've gotten, aim to lift 5–15 pounds more weight for every exercise each week.

Mistake to Avoid:

Don't overdo it. Everyone needs a break from their workout routine—even Olympic athletes. Overtraining can lead to muscle aches and tears, joint injuries, fatigue, decreased immunity, and even depression. You can take as long as a week off from your routine without significantly reducing your fitness level.

Lift three times per week, taking a day off between sessions. Do *Workout One* on Mondays and Fridays, and *Workout Two* on Wednesdays. To extend the program beyond our four-week starter program, continue to add weight, and cycle through reps as described above. Take a week or two off to recover after every ten weeks of training.

Begin each workout with 5–10 minutes of light aerobic activity of your choice (preferably one that works both your upper and lower body). At the end of the workout, stretch all the major muscle groups used (see "The Sexy Side of Stretching," page 43).

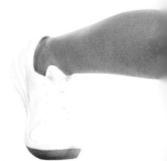

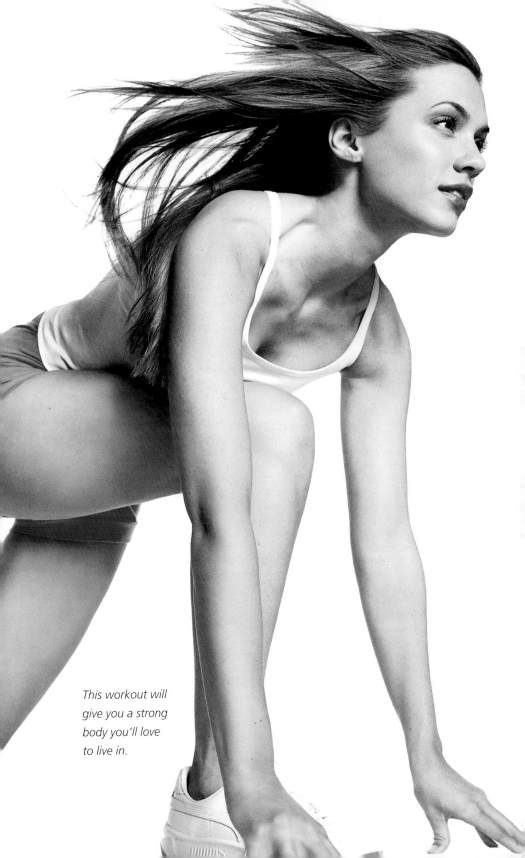

This workout will give you a strong body you'll love to live in.

workout one: monday and friday

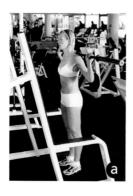
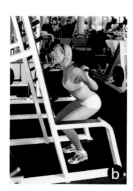

1. Barbell Squat. *Put a bar on a rack and stand so that the bar rests across your upper back, feet hip-width apart and legs straight (not locked). Hold the bar with an overhand grip, hands a little more than hip-width apart. Lift the bar. Contract your abs as you drop your tailbone toward the floor (a). Keeping body weight over your heels, bend knees and lower hips until your thighs are almost parallel to the floor (b). Straighten your legs; do reps. Strengthens quadriceps, hamstrings, and buttocks. Starting weight: 45–65 pounds.*

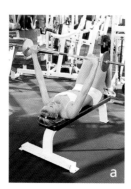
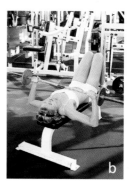

2. Barbell Bench Press. *Lie on a flat bench, heels on the edge of bench. Hold the bar overhand, hands slightly more than shoulder-width apart. Lift the bar and hold it over your midchest, arms straight (not locked). Contract abs to sup-port back (a). Keeping wrists in line with elbows, inhale as you slowly lower bar toward your chest. Bend your arms and lower the bar until elbows are in line with shoulders (b). Exhale as you press bar back up; do reps. Strengthens chest, front shoulders, and triceps. Starting weight: 35–45 pounds.*

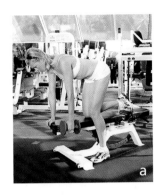 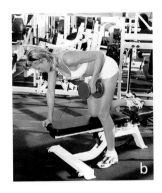

3. One-Arm Row. Put your right knee and right hand on a flat bench, knee in line with your hip, hand just in front of right shoulder. Hold a dumbbell in left hand, then bend forward from your hips so your back is parallel to the floor. Let left arm hang down, palm facing in and in line with shoulder (a). Contract back muscles and keep shoulder blades back as you pull weight toward your waist without rotating hips or shoulders (b). Straighten arm, do reps, switch sides and repeat with right arm for all reps. Strengthens middle back, rear shoulders, and some biceps. Starting weight: 10–20 pounds.

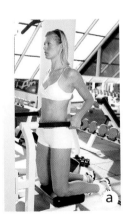 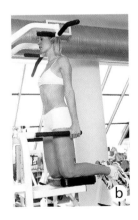

4. Tri-Dip. Stand or kneel on an assisted tri-dip machine. Put hands on lower bars directly under your shoulders, bending arms to 45 degrees (a). Press up by straightening elbows (don't lock them) (b). Slowly return to starting position; do reps. Strengthens triceps. Starting weight: Begin with assistance at 50–65 percent of your body weight (about 65–80 pounds for a 130-pound woman).

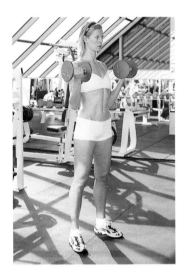

5. Dumbbell Curl. *Hold dumbbells and stand with feet hip-width apart, arms hanging by your sides, palms facing forward. Contract your abs. Keeping elbows lined up under your shoulders, bend your arms and lift dumbbells up and in toward your shoulders. Lower; do reps. Strengthens biceps. Starting weight: 5–10 pounds in each hand.*

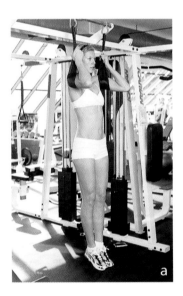
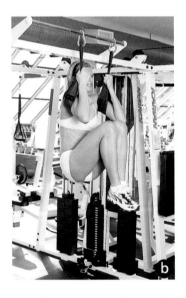

6. Hanging Crunch *Attach two hanging straps from the center hooks of a double-cable pulley machine. Standing on a stool if needed, put your upper arms through straps and let legs hang straight down so your body forms a straight line (a). Without swinging legs, use abs to bend knees up to hip height. Contract abs more to curl your pelvis up toward your ribs with knees bent (b). Slowly return to starting position; do reps. Strengthens abdominals. No added weight.*

workout two: wednesdays

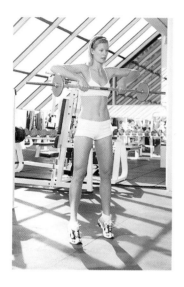

1a. High Pull. *Stand, feet hip-width apart, arms straight, bar resting at thigh height, abs tight, back in neutral position. Bend knees slightly to lower bar to just below your kneecaps; bend elbows to pull the bar up as high as you can (between your waist and your chest) as you straighten your legs and lift yourself up onto your toes. Keeping bar in close, slowly lower it to thigh height; do reps. Strengthens hamstrings, quadriceps, middle shoulder, midback, and biceps. Starting weight: 25–45 pounds for three sets. When you can lift 65–75 pounds easily, switch to a Dead Lift.*

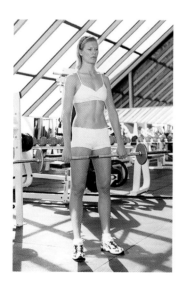

1b. Dead Lift. *Stand with feet hip-width apart, knees bent, holding a barbell at shin height (not shown). Straighten legs to a full standing position, keeping bar close to thighs. Bend knees, lowering bar; do reps. Strengthens buttocks, hamstrings, and back extensors. Starting weight: 65–95 pounds.*

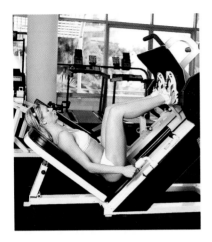

2. Leg Press. *Lie on a leg-press machine adjusted to a 45-degree angle. Put feet in the center of the plate, hip-width apart, legs straight (not shown). Contract abs to brace back against seat back. Release handle locks; keeping weight toward heels, bend knees to form 90-degree angles. Straighten legs, pressing plate away from you; repeat for reps. Strengthens quadriceps, buttocks, and hamstrings. Starting weight: 100–135 pounds.*

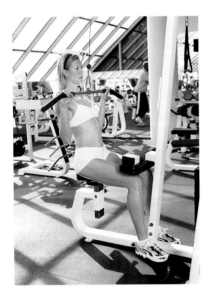

3. Lat Pull-Down. *Attach a long bar to a high pulley machine. Hold the bar overhand, hands slightly more than shoulder-width apart. Sit with thighs under rollers, knees bent, and feet flat. With arms straight, lean slightly back from your hips so bar hangs right over your chest, arms straight (not shown). Squeeze shoulder blades back and down as you bend elbows toward the floor; lift chest to meet the bar. Slowly straighten arms; do reps. Strengthens middle back, rear shoulders, and some biceps. Starting weight: 40–60 pounds.*

4. Incline Press *(not shown). Repeat the Barbell Bench Press* (Workout One) *on an incline bench adjusted to 30 degrees. Starting weight: 25–45 pounds.*

5. Tri-Dip *(see* Workout One*).*

6. Dumbbell Curl *(see* Workout One*).*

7. Crunch *(not shown). Lie face up with feet on a bench, knees bent and fingertips behind your head. Use your abs to curl upper torso off the bench. To progress, do this holding a 10–25-pound weight plate on your chest. Strengthens abdominals.*

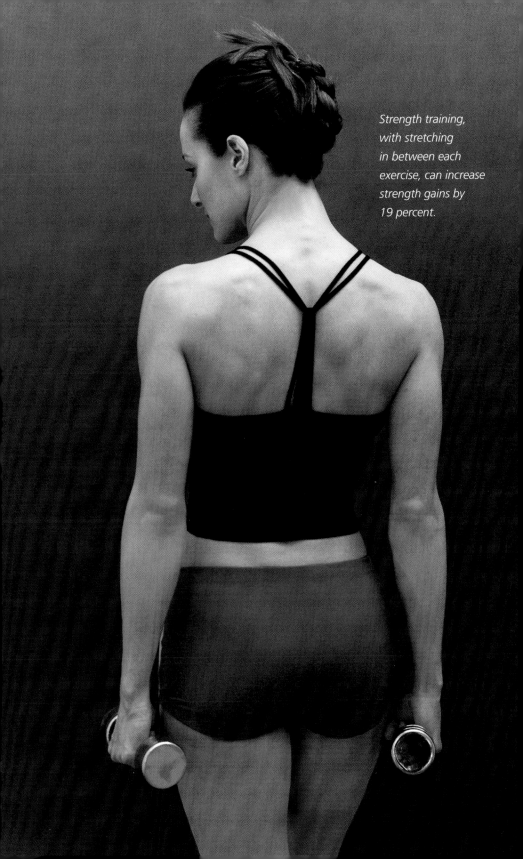

Strength training, with stretching in between each exercise, can increase strength gains by 19 percent.

pumping up your strength training

Research has shown that people who repeatedly perform the same training routine tend to plateau after 4–6 months. When you find yourself sleepwalking through that same weight-machine circuit without seeing any additional progress in your muscle tone or strength, it's time to tweak your routine. Here are some techniques to make your weight workouts more effective and fun.

- *Split the routine.* If you usually train all of your muscle groups in a single workout session, split up your routine so you work your upper and lower body on different days. You'll likely hit each muscle group longer and harder.

- *Progressing.* Regularly increase weight and change your number of reps. For example, start with one set of 10–12 reps for 4 weeks, then do 2 sets of 8–10 reps the next 4 weeks, then 3 sets of 6–8 reps for the next 4 weeks. Increase weight as you decrease reps. It's effective and will keep you alert.

- *"Breakdown" training.* After tiring out your muscles at 10 reps, immediately reduce the weight (by 10–20 percent) and squeeze out 2–4 more reps. You reach deeper when your muscles are already fatigued. Only do this for 8 weeks, and then return to more moderate workouts for four weeks to avoid injury.

- *Heavier weights.* If you can easily complete 12 reps, go heavier. You'll plateau when your muscles get used to a weight.

- *Periodization.* Create 4–6-week training periods. Vary your exercises for each muscle group for each period. Instead of doing the same flat-bench dumbbell chest press, try performing a chest press on an incline or decline bench. Use a barbell instead of dumbbells. Focus on strength for 4 weeks by lifting heavier weights for 6–8 reps; overall strength and endurance with 8–12 repetitions. The possibilities are almost limitless, and when you lift different loads and do new exercises to work your muscles from different angles, you reach different fibers and stimulate more growth.

- *"Pre-exhaust" training.* Challenge each muscle group by first doing an isolation exercise. Then without resting, do a multimuscle move that also works your chosen muscle group. For instance, for a killer quad workout, do 10 reps on the leg-extension machine and then a set of 10 reps on the leg press. For your triceps, do triceps extensions followed by a chest press. You'll reach more muscle fibers. (Do for 6–8 weeks.)

- *Slow down.* Take a full 10 seconds to lift the weight and 4 seconds to lower it. This forces you to rely on muscle strength, not momentum. This can boost your strength 50 percent more than the traditional 2 seconds up, 4 seconds down. Do only 4–6 repetitions per set and limit this rigorous training to 6–8 weeks, then go back to an 8–12-rep program to recover.

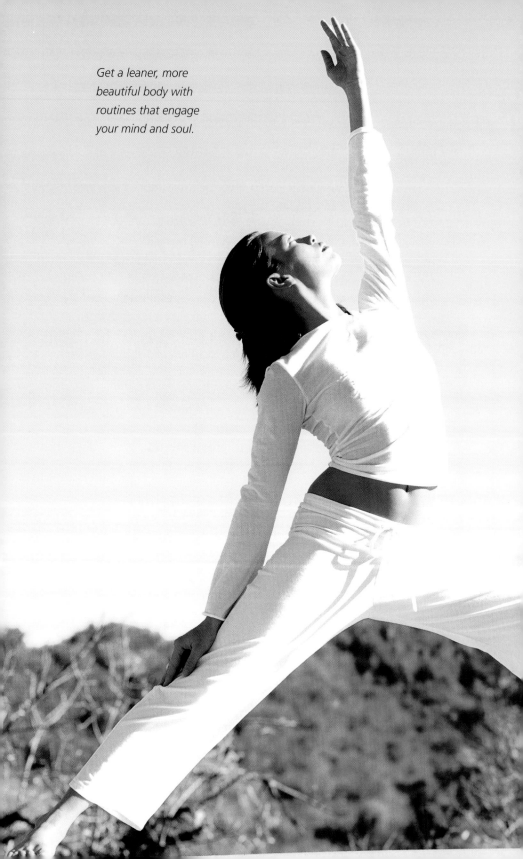

Get a leaner, more beautiful body with routines that engage your mind and soul.

the mind-body workout

Whether you've hit a plateau in your fitness program, think that your routine lacks balance, or don't feel energized after exercising, you can transform your routine by exercising *mindfully*. This is not as esoteric as it sounds. Mindfulness simply means being conscious and receptive to the present moment. It means paying attention to each experience so it doesn't pass us by. We're often so focused on what's coming next that we miss out on what's happening right now. By directing our mind to the present, we live real *moments,* rather than worrying about ones that may never transpire.

Working out is a classic example of how we tend to focus on the future. Many of us ignore how our body feels when we exercise. We distract ourselves by reading a magazine on the treadmill or thinking about what we're going to do when we go home. But our workouts can improve dramatically when we do activities that put us in tune with our body.

Any exercise can be mindful, but probably the most popular workout for connecting mind and body is yoga. You may be surprised to find out what an incredible workout yoga can be—deep breathing combined with fluid movement and challenging poses can work your heart and lungs, tone your muscles, and leave you feeling clearheaded and alert.

In this program designed by *Shape*® fitness editor Linda Shelton, you'll move smoothly from one pose to the next— a progression, or flow, known as a *vinyasa,* rather than holding each position. In addition to the cardiovascular calorie-burn this achieves, you'll help tone and reshape your entire body, making you look longer, stronger, and leaner. At the same time, you'll increase flexibility and balance.

the plan

Do these moves in the order shown at least 3 times a week. To make it a truly cardio-style yoga workout, move from one pose to the next without stopping (but also without getting breathless), giving yourself 4–6 counts to move into each pose before going on to the next. The first week, repeat the sequence 5 times; add an additional repetition each week until by week 4 you're doing 8 repetitions.

Warm up by moving slowly through the first sequence of moves, giving yourself 6–8 counts for each pose.

Before you begin each pose, inhale—filling lungs, ribs, and belly—then exhale slowly and smoothly as you move into position. Don't rush; keep both inhale and exhale even and equal in length.

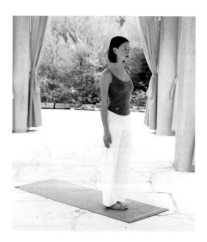

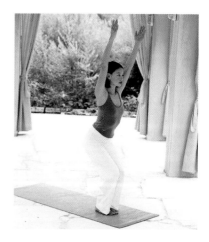

1. Mountain Pose. *Stand with big toes together, heels slightly apart, legs straight, and abs tight with arms at sides.*

2. Chair Pose. *Keeping knees and feet together, bend both knees, weight back into heels as if sitting in a chair. Extend arms overhead, palms facing in and shoulders down.*

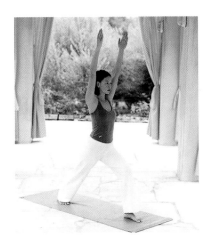

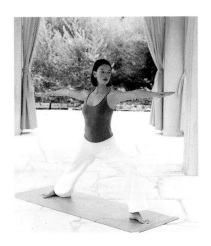

3. *Warrior I.* *From Chair Pose, straighten legs and take a large step back with your right foot, keeping hips square and toes pointing forward. Bend left knee over left ankle, keeping right leg straight, keeping arms extended overhead, alongside your ears, palms facing inward.*

4. *Warrior II.* *From Warrior I, turn hips to the side and rotate back foot as you lower both arms to shoulder height, palms down. (Separate feet a little farther if necessary to keep front knee bent directly over ankle.) Turn head to look over middle fingers of left hand, which is extending straight in front of you.*

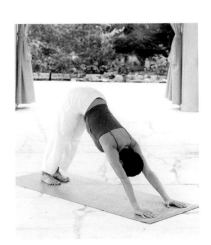

5. Downward-Facing Dog. *From Warrior II, turn toes of right foot forward aligned with left foot; bend forward from hips, pressing hands on floor on each side of left foot just in front of shoulders. Step left foot back to meet right; lift hips to form an inverted V.*

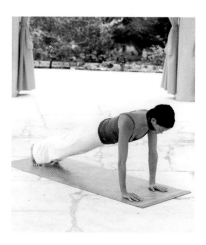

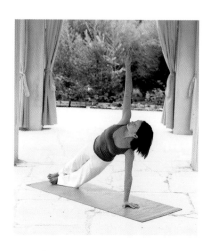

6. Plank Pose. *From Downward-Facing Dog, lower hips until body forms one straight line from head to heels. Use abs to keep torso from collapsing toward floor.*

7. Side Plank Pose. *From Plank Pose, squeeze feet together and roll to outer edge of left foot. Keeping feet stacked, legs straight, with left hand directly under left shoulder, arms straight and shoulders drawn back, lift right arm to open body and look up at right hand.*

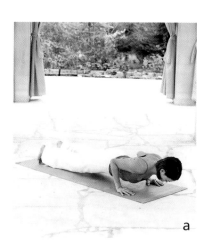

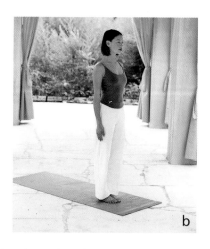

a

b

8. Chatarunga. *Return to Plank Pose, then keep abs tight and bend elbows to lower entire body toward floor as far as you can without rounding shoulders forward, lifting butt up, or letting hips sag. Lower all the way to the floor (a), then push back to Downward-Facing Dog, walk feet forward, bend knees, and roll up to Mountain Pose (b).*

major muscle groups

We've told you repeatedly to stretch the major muscle groups. So what are they? There's nothing too technical about it—you probably already know them by their familiar names.

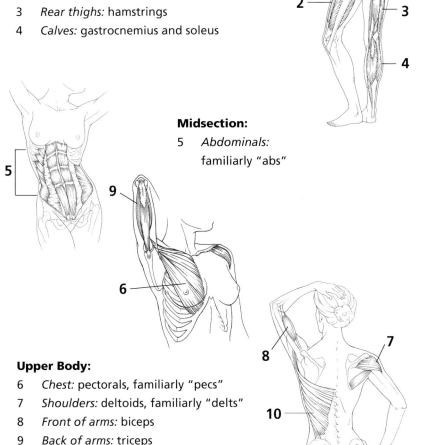

Lower Body:

1   *Buttocks:* gluteal muscles, familiarly "glutes"
2   *Front thighs:* quadriceps, familiarly "quads"
3   *Rear thighs:* hamstrings
4   *Calves:* gastrocnemius and soleus

Midsection:

5   *Abdominals:* familiarly "abs"

Upper Body:

6   *Chest:* pectorals, familiarly "pecs"
7   *Shoulders:* deltoids, familiarly "delts"
8   *Front of arms:* biceps
9   *Back of arms:* triceps
10 *Back:* Latissimus dorsi, familiarly "lats"

stretching glossary

There's more than one way to lengthen your muscles. Here are some terms you may come across in books, classes, and videos.

Active stretching. Also referred to as active-isolated stretching (AIS), this involves elongating your target muscle by contracting the opposing muscle. For example, to stretch your hamstrings, you'd tighten the muscles in the front of your thigh as you lengthen the muscles in the back of the thigh. The tension in your quadriceps inhibits tension in the hamstrings, which gives you a better stretch. Active stretches are often very hard for more than a few seconds.

Dynamic stretching. This involves some sort of repeated, short-duration movement, such as leg swings, arm swings, toe touches, or torso twists, which take you to the edge of your range of motion. The intensity may range from low (a gentle motion without any bouncing or "jerking") to high (faster and more forceful motion), which is only appropriate for sports-specific or more intense activities. You should only do this type of stretching under the supervision of a qualified personal trainer or a physical therapist.

Static stretching. This is a lower-intensity, longer-duration method that involves slowly moving to the edge of your range of motion and then staying there for an extended period of time (preferably at least 20–30 seconds). The stretches in this workout are static—but you can make them dynamic by adding some movement: Take 2 counts to move into each stretch, hold the position for 4 counts, then release it in 2 counts; repeat the sequence 3–5 times.

the sexy side of stretching

As you've seen, all four *Shape Your Life* workouts incorporate stretching. That's because diligent stretching is as important as strength training and cardiovascular workouts in terms of fitness gains. But in case you're thinking of stretching as a disposable part of a "real" workout, think again. Stretching has become one of the hottest fitness trends sweeping the country. Gyms are even getting creative, with stretching classes that include candlelight and aromatherapy. Flexibility workouts have gotten a face-lift—and are helping devotees everywhere look and feel longer, stronger, and sexier.

There's a good reason why stretching is so popular. It can give your muscles a more elongated look while improving posture and range of motion, boosting your energy, and increasing your mental focus. "Boosting your flexibility can help prevent postural imbalances that can cause hip and back pain, and relieve muscle tension that can lead to feeling tired," says Deborah Ellison, a licensed physical therapist and owner of Advanced Personal Training Institute in Memphis.

We asked Ellison to create a stretching workout that feels as good as it makes you look. These six stretches are designed to lengthen the major muscle groups that tend to be tight in many people. While you don't need fancy equipment for this elongation workout, a few optional props—namely, a broomstick or dowel, a chair, a towel, a book (about one to two inches thick) and a yoga strap or bathrobe tie—can be beneficial. These tools will keep you honest and help you work safely and effectively within your range of motion.

Quick Tip: *Keep a training log. "Write down everything you can—the course, your time, your pace, who you worked out with," says running coach Mindy Solkin. Also note the details of your strength workouts. Then, use your log to see which training patterns and techniques seem to work best for you and which ones seem to lead to excessive fatigue, injuries, or plateaus.*

"If you're trying to do a stretch that's too hard for you, your muscles will tense up instead of relaxing and lengthening," says Ellison. And props aren't just for beginners. As you improve, you may need to use them differently, but they can be beneficial no matter how advanced you are.

Conscious, controlled breathing is also key to getting the most out of this or any stretching program. "A lot of the benefits we attribute to stretching are actually a result of mindful breathing," says Ellison. "Long inhalations and exhalations can help bring your mind into the movement, relax your muscles, and make you aware of where you're holding your tension. As you do each stretch, think about how your body feels, and don't force it. This should be a soothing, delicious experience—not hurried or painful."

the plan

While you should incorporate these stretches into your strength-training and aerobic activities, you can improve your results by doing them on your days off. Do the following stretches in the order listed. Inhale slowly (at least 4 counts) through your nose. Sink into your stretch as you exhale slowly (at least 4 counts) through your nose or mouth. Hold each stretch for 3–5 breaths (about 20–40 seconds) without bouncing. Try to take each stretch to the edge of discomfort, but ease off if you feel pain.

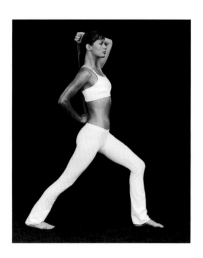

1. Goddess Lunge. *Stand with your feet hip-width apart, then take a big step forward with your left foot, keeping your right foot flat on the floor. Hold a long dowel, broom handle, or stretch cord vertically behind your back with your left hand behind your head, palm facing inward, and your right hand at the base of your spine, thumb pointing up. Keeping right foot flat on the floor and torso erect, bend left knee into a lunge, with left knee above left ankle. Keep torso lifted and shoulders back. Hold for 3–5 breaths (about 20–40 seconds), then release. Switch hands and feet, then repeat. Stretches hip flexors, quadriceps, front shoulder, and upper chest.*

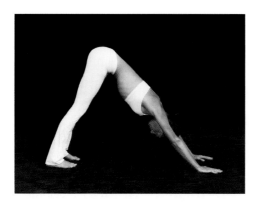

2. Downward-Facing Dog. *Stand with feet hip-width apart, toes turned in slightly, heels on the floor. Keeping legs as straight as possible (bend knees slightly, if necessary), bend forward from your hips, and place hands on the floor so your body forms an inverted V. (If you're new to this challeng-ing move or if your calves and hamstrings feel tight, stand with your heels on a book.) Keeping arms straight, press your sitting bones (bottom of your buttocks) up toward the ceiling. Stay here for 3–5 breaths, lengthening your spine as you inhale and sinking into the stretch as you exhale. Stretches shoulders, hamstrings, and spine.*

3. Lying Torso Twist. *Lie on your left side, with hips and knees bent at 90-degree angles and stacked on top of one another. To keep head in a neutral position, you may want to rest it on a rolled towel. Extend both arms in front of you at chest height, palms together (a). Inhale as you lift your right arm up and over to your right side, then exhale as you lay it on the floor at shoulder height, palm up.*

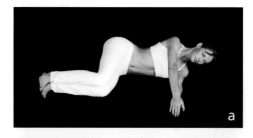

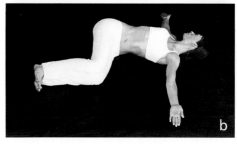

Keep your eyes on your arm as you extend it over your head, and then turn head to the right as your stretch (b). Only rotate as far as your can while keeping knees and hips stacked. Stay here for 3–5 breaths, then switch to right side and repeat the twist in the opposite direction. Stretches front of shoulders and chest, intercostal muscles (between ribs), and obliques. Strengthens spine extensors and rotators.

4. Lying Hamstring Stretch. *Lie face up on the floor with both legs extended straight. Holding a strap or bathrobe tie in both hands, bend right knee in toward your chest and place the strap around your right arch. Extend right leg straight up in the air so it's in line with your right hip (a). Keeping left leg on the floor, toes pointed, inhale, then exhale and use the strap to bring your right leg toward your face: hold for 3–5 breaths, then release. Grasp both ends of the strap with your left hand, then bring right leg toward your left shoulder*

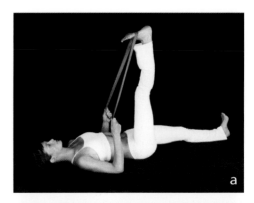

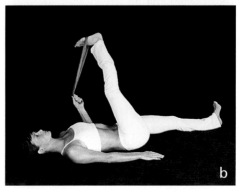

(shown); holding the stretch for 3–5 breaths (b). Repeat, using right hand to bring leg toward right shoulder. Switch the stretch to the left leg and repeat. Stretches all three hamstring muscles, iliotibial band (on outside of thigh), and hip adductors of raised leg as well as hip flexors of the leg on floor.

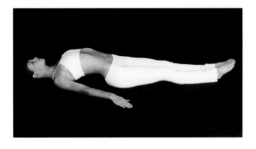

5. Rib Lift. *Lie faceup on the floor, legs straight, arms relaxed by your sides. Keeping your head, shoulders, and buttocks on the floor, arch your spine, lifting it up as if to open the spaces between your vertebrae. Your back will come up off the floor. Hold this stretch for 3–5 breaths, then release. Stretches intercostals muscles, front shoulders, and front rotator muscles; also activates back extensors.*

the program in action

A bond trader and mother of two young children, Mary Knobler began her day before dawn and barely had a minute to breathe before collapsing into bed at night. She was hardly overweight (at 130 pounds on a 5' 3" frame) but didn't exercise and wanted to be in better physical shape; she often felt lethargic. But she was convinced that there was no time for exercise in her hectic life. "When I came home from work, I didn't want to be away from my kids. I couldn't do it," she recalls.

Then Knobler joined a gym a year after the birth of her second child. She began swimming, an activity she'd loved as a kid. She found herself enjoying exercise rather than seeing it as a means to whip her body into shape. "It felt really good to be in the water again. Something clicked, and it was no longer 'Should I exercise or shouldn't I?'—I was going swimming," she says.

Exercise quickly became a routine part of Knobler's life, as basic as brushing her teeth. She swims immediately after work or during her kids' nap time (when she used to need a nap herself). Some days, she'll strap the kids into the baby jogger, leash up the family dog, and take a three- to five-mile run. She also lifts free weights and jumps rope—anything that fits into her day. Today, at 109 pounds with her body-fat composition in check, she sings a very different tune: "Not only can I do it, I have much more energy for everything."

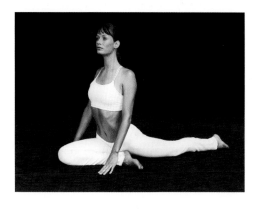

6. Modified Pigeon.

Begin on all fours, arms straight and hands in line with your shoulders. Bend your right knee to bring your right foot forward (if you're tight and you need it, place a rolled towel under your left hip). Extend left leg behind you and rotate your hips so they're square and facing forward. Walk your hands slightly forward, keeping arms straight, and "puff" up your chest, keeping length in your spine. Stay here for 3–5 breaths, then switch legs and repeat. Stretches posterior hip, hip flexor, upper torso, and spine extensors.

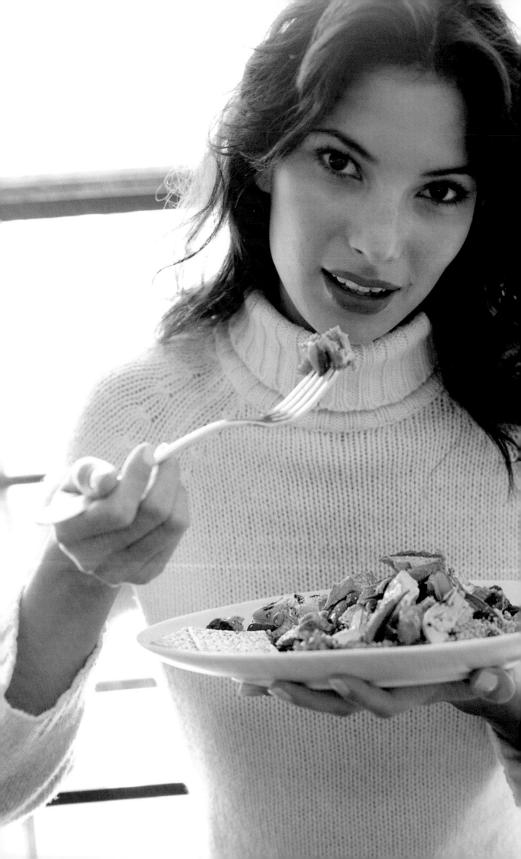

chapter two
your diet

Quick Tip: *Even when you're dining alone, make your meal special. You're less likely to overeat if you set a place at the table and concentrate on enjoying the flavors, colors, and textures of your food. Other ideas for mindful eating include: decorating your table with flowers and candles; listening to slow, quiet music; and saying a prayer or personal affirmation to express your gratitude for your meal.*

what you'll learn

Shape's approach to nutrition is to help you create a lifestyle eating plan based on adding satisfying and delicious foods to your diet, and also to understand what to eat more of to become leaner and healthier. Using this chapter, you'll follow the *Shape*® Food Pyramid and Plan every day, so you'll:

- eat eight or more servings of vegetables and fruits
- consume the equivalent of nine cups of water
- eat at least six servings of whole grains
- eat fish and legumes (mostly beans and peas) for at least one of three healthy protein sources
- choose healthy fats (from olive and canola oils, nuts, seeds, and fish) in moderation

- consume three high-calcium foods, including one nondairy source
- eat more often (no less than every four hours!)
- get enough calories—at least 1,800 a day
- fill your plate at every meal with vegetables and whole grains, and small portions of protein and fat

how you'll do it

When *Shape®* says "diet," we don't mean an imposed regimen of deprivation. We want you to enjoy nature's bounty in all its infinite variety. Before we tell you more about the *Shape®* Food Pyramid and Plan, though, it will help to know a little bit about how the experts define a healthy eating regimen. The basic standard is the government's Food Guide Pyramid, designed by the U.S. Department of Agriculture (USDA) about a decade ago. The pyramid has at its base six to eleven daily servings of bread, cereal, rice, and pasta. Next up, five to nine daily servings of fruits and vegetables. Atop that, two to three daily servings of dairy products, and the same number of servings of meat, poultry, fish, dry beans, eggs, or nuts. Finally, at the peak, fats, oils, and sweets used sparingly.

Mistake to Avoid: *The quickest way to throw your healthy eating plan off track? Skip breakfast! Not eating a morning meal sets you up for bingeing later in the day. Start the day with a mix of carbs and protein and you'll stay satisfied until your midmorning snack.*

Since the USDA published its Food Pyramid, however, many nutritionists have argued that it doesn't reflect the latest research and could inadvertently promote a diet filled with saturated fat, which is linked to heart disease and cancer. As a result, various other nutritional authorities at universities and health-related foundations have created competing nutrition structures, including a Mediterranean diet pyramid, two different vegetarian pyramids, a Latin American pyramid, a Native American pyramid, an Indian pyramid, and several Asian pyramids.

what's your diet IQ?

Been on more diets than you can count? Then you know that practice does not make perfect. In fact, it usually makes your eating habits worse. Diets don't work, and many are based on myths that are counterproductive. To find your dietary pitfalls, take this quiz designed by Nancy Clark, M.S., R.D., a leading sports nutritionist. Answer each question honestly, yes or no, to find out what mistakes you commonly make.

YES NO

___ ___ 1. I get on track by eating a light breakfast.

___ ___ 2. I try to stay away from bread. In fact, I rarely eat bagels for breakfast or sandwiches for lunch anymore.

___ ___ 3. I'm too busy to eat lunch. Besides, skipping meals is a good way to save calories.

___ ___ 4. I crave sweets daily and fight the temptation to eat sugar.

___ ___ 5. I try not to snack. It's better to save your appetite for real meals.

___ ___ 6. I save calories from breakfast and lunch so I can eat a bigger dinner.

___ ___ 7. I've stopped having pasta, potatoes, or other carbohydrates with dinner.

___ ___ 8. I find myself eating too much junk after 8 P.M.

___ ___ 9. I allow myself one "cheat day" per week, when I eat what I truly crave.

___ ___ 10. A girl can't get enough protein. Could Jennifer and Brad (and those other celebrity *Zoners*) all be wrong?

SCORING

If you answered yes to questions 1, 3, 4, 6, or 8, you seem to perceive food as being the fattening enemy and put lots of effort into trying not to eat—that is, until you succumb to extreme hunger. Make peace with food and embrace it as healthy and life-sustaining.

If you answered yes to questions 4, 5, and 8, you're dieting "too hard" and restricting your calorie intake too much. You need to nourish yourself with healthful foods high in nutrients rather than "empty calories," and curb your craving for sweets.

If you answered yes to questions 2, 4, 7, 9, or 10, you try to eliminate too many of your favorite foods. No foods are taboo, and you can lose weight and still enjoy your must-haves (whether it's pizza, chocolate, even cheesecake) in moderation.

usda

fats, oils, sweets: use sparingly

milk, yogurt, cheese: 2–3 servings	meat, poultry, fish, dry beans, eggs, nuts: 2–3 servings

vegetables: 3–5 servings	fruit: 2–4 servings

bread, cereal, rice, pasta: 6–11 servings

mediterranean

red meat	a few times per month
sweets	
eggs	
poultry	a few times per week
fish	
cheese & yogurt	
olive oil	wine in moderatio

fruits	beans, legumes, nuts	vegetables

bread, rice, pasta, couscous, polenta, bulgur, other grains & potatoes   daily

The USDA Pyramid. This pyramid fails to distinguish between refined and whole grains, whole and low-fat dairy products, and disease-causing and healthy fats. It also lumps together meat, fish, legumes, eggs, and nuts, when these foods are far from equally healthy. Technically, this plan permits three glasses of whole milk and a half pound of high-fat hamburger per day!

The Mediterranean Pyramid. This pyramid gets high marks for highlighting olive oil, fish, and legumes. But it implies that you should get all your fat from olive oil when, in fact, you need some of the nutrients in other oil sources such as canola, flaxseed, and walnuts. It, too, doesn't stipulate whole grains and doesn't give daily serving ranges. The "alcohol in moderation" recommendation is controversial.

The Loma Linda Vegetarian Pyramid. This pyramid does specify whole grains and daily serving ranges. It includes eggs, but considers dairy optional, with no mention of fortified soy milk as a replacement.

loma linda vegetarian

limit sweets

dairy: 2–3 servings	eggs: 0–4 servings a week
	optional

vegetable oils: 0–4 servings   daily

nuts and seeds: 0–2 servings

fruits: at least 2 servings	vegetables: at least 4 servings

whole grains: 8–11 servings	legumes: at least 1 serving

the Shape® *food pyramid*

The *Shape*® Food Pyramid combines the best aspects of these models while including important features not currently found in any of them. For instance, we add water to our version. Research reveals that most Americans don't consume nearly as much fluid as they need. In the short term, if you're not drinking enough, you may feel tired, edgy, slightly headachy, and eventually thirsty. In the long term, mild dehydration can increase the risk of a number of diseases.

Also, we specifically recommend avoiding trans fatty acids, which are significant contributors to heart disease. They are found in many prepackaged and fast foods.

The *Shape*® pyramid also differentiates between poultry breast and other, fattier parts of the bird; separates whole and refined grains; and is specific about types of oils. Lest it seem like there are a lot of specifications, don't worry—we don't ban chocolate or insist that you eat broccoli at every meal. Our priority is good health, and our recommendations are based on studies that show which eating patterns are likely to reduce your risk of disease. However, we strongly believe that an optimal diet includes a variety of foods—one that makes eating a pleasure. The emphasis of our smart eating plan is good health. A great collateral reward is fat loss and weight maintenance.

We also believe that physical activity is a crucial part of the smart way to stay healthy. Our food pyramid goes hand-in-hand with our exercise program (see Chapter One for training details).

the key to healthy eating

The following is a key to our food pyramid, from the bottom up, including serving sizes and the rationale behind our choices.

First tier: Eight or more servings a day of vegetables and fruits—especially those of darker colors, since they tend to contain the most phytochemicals (protective chemicals found naturally in plant foods). A serving can be fresh, frozen, dried, canned, and in some cases, juiced.

the SHAPE® food pyramid

the SHAPE® exercise pyramid

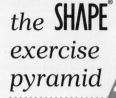

trans fatty acids, saturated fats, alcohol
Limit or avoid

red meat, poultry (other than breast meat)
No more than 3–4 servings a month

salad dressings, mayo, and vegetable oils (i.e., polyunsaturated fats)
No more than 4–5 servings a week

| eggs No more than 4–5 servings a week | skinless breast meat of poultry No more than 4–5 servings a week | refined low-fat grains No more than 4–5 servings a week |

strength training twice a week

stretching daily

cardio exercise (at least 30 mins. daily)

optional

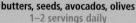

olive oil, canola oil, nuts, nut butters, seeds, avocados, olives
1–2 servings daily

legumes
1–2 servings daily

fish (if you don't eat fish, eat walnuts or flaxseed to get omega-3 fatty acids)
3–4 servings a week

milk, milk products (primarily plain, nonfat) and/or calcium- and vitamin D-fortified soy milk
3 servings daily

whole grains
6 or more servings daily

water
9 or more servings daily

vegetables and fruits (fresh, frozen, dried, and some juices)
8 or more servings daily

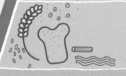

Serving size: 1 piece of fruit, 1 cup raw, ½ cup canned or cooked, 1 ounce dried, 6 ounces juice.

Rationale: Eat as wide a variety of fresh fruits and vegetables as possible (or canned when fresh produce is limited). Hundreds of studies document the disease-preventing benefits associated with high fruit and vegetable intake. Remember, though, that not all juices are created equal. Apple and white grape juices are virtually devoid of nutrients, whereas orange juice and tomato juice are rich in vitamin C and phytochemicals.

Second tier: 9 or more servings a day of water or its equivalent. Fruits, vegetables, and other liquids in foods contribute about 1 liter (roughly 4 cups) a day.

Serving size: 1 cup.

Rationale: How much water you need depends on how much you exercise. For active women, 9 cups is generally not enough. If you're sufficiently hydrated, your urine should be clear and plentiful, not dark yellow and sparse.

Third tier: 6 or more servings a day of whole grains.

Serving size: 1 slice bread; ½ English muffin; ½ hamburger bun; ½ bagel; 1 tortilla; ½ cup of cooked pasta, rice, or cereal; 1 ounce ready-to-eat cereal.

Rationale: Americans are dreadfully low in this crucial high-fiber, nutrient-dense category. As much as possible, choose whole-grain cereals over more-processed varieties, and whole-wheat bread over refined breads. Breads made from refined flour contain minimal nutrients and virtually no fiber.

Fourth tier: 3 servings a day of primarily plain, nonfat milk and milk products; calcium and vitamin-D fortified soy milk, tofu, cereal, or orange juice; or calcium-rich foods such as canned salmon.

Serving size: 1 cup milk, 1 ounce fortified cheese, 1 cup yogurt, 1 cup soy milk or orange juice, 1 cup of fortified cereal, 3 ounces of tofu, 3 ounces of fish.

Rationale: Milk products are excellent sources of calcium, but even reduced-fat (2 percent) milk is high in saturated fat. Choose low-fat (1 percent) or nonfat (skimmed) varieties as much as possible. Also, minimize flavored yogurts, which are often high in sugar. Make sure soy milk is calcium enriched, although it needn't be nonfat since its fat isn't saturated.

did someone say chocolate?

Okay, we did say you didn't have to give up chocolate, didn't we? If you ignore your intense yen for it, you could become fixated and end up overindulging. Besides, chocolate contains polyphenols, the same heart-friendly antioxidants found in red wine and green tea. One-third of its fat is stearic acid, which doesn't raise cholesterol. Another third consists of monounsaturated oleic acid, which actually reduces cholesterol.

But chocolate's calories can add up fast, so stick with treats that contain cocoa butter or chocolate liqueur. Get your fix by adding powdered cocoa to skim milk, from a chocolate-flavored calcium chew, or from a low-fat treat such as a Fudgesicle. If nothing but the real thing will do, have two miniature (0.7-ounce) candy bars. They offer instant portion control, assuming you can refrain from eating the entire bag. Or indulge in one fine piece of chocolate, being sure to factor it into your calorie and fat allowance.

"I allow myself to enjoy Godiva chocolate every day," says *Shape*® reader Lee Ann Hatcher of Springfield, Illinois. "Just one piece of the very best chocolate in the world is better than any cheaper candy bar that I've ever tried. I savor every bite, and I don't feel guilty." Chocolate lovers are in for more treats in the future: There's a growing trend for specialty chocolatiers to introduce darker and less sweet cocoa beans with as much variety as wines and coffees.

the whole (grain) story

Why all this fuss about whole grains? One reason is that it's rich in fiber, and fiber has many attributes.

1. It curbs overeating. According to the American Dietetic Association, fiber-full foods are a natural appetite suppressant. They take up more room in your stomach than other foods, so you feel full faster. Fiber is slower to digest, so it keeps hunger at bay longer. And most fiber-rich foods simply take more time to chew (think granola versus doughnuts), so your brain has more time to register that you've had enough before you've had too much.

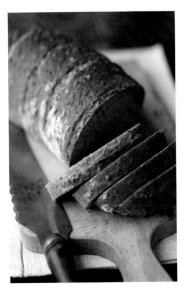

2. It whisks away calories. Because most fiber leaves the body undigested, the calories in fiber-rich foods are less accessible to the body. USDA studies reveal that for each gram of fiber you eat, you absorb about seven fewer calories from food. (And speaking of "whisking," fiber is your body's broom. Insoluble fiber binds with water to usher waste out of the body smoothly and dependably.)

3. It cuts the fat. Fiber-rich foods are naturally low in fat. For instance, you can save 17 grams of fat by eating a cup of kidney beans instead of a half cup of refined macaroni and cheese.

4. Its sources are nutrient-dense. Most fruits and vegetables are packed with vitamins, and whole-grain breads and cereals are fortified with lots of good stuff, including folic acid, a B vitamin that plays a fundamental role in the growth and reproduction of cells and is especially needed by all women of childbearing age to prevent birth defects. Other important nutrients include magnesium, copper, and zinc.

5. It has numerous health benefits. Various studies show that a fiber-rich diet might lower harmful LDL cholesterol, possibly reducing heart-disease and diabetes risk.

Fifth tier: 1–2 servings a day of legumes such as chickpeas, lentils, or soybeans. 3–4 servings a week of fish.

Serving size: ¾ cup cooked legumes. 3 ounces of fish.

Rationale: Legumes are high in protein, free of saturated fats, and packed with disease-protective nutrients and fiber. Fish oils, a.k.a. omega-3 fatty acids, appear to lower the risk of heart disease and may even help prevent breast cancer. If you don't eat fish, be sure to consume flaxseed or walnuts—they contain linolenic acid, a precursor to omega-3 that appears to have similar benefits.

Sixth tier: 1–2 servings a day of olive or canola oil, nut butters, nuts, seeds, olives, or avocado.

Serving size: 1 tablespoon of oil, 1 tablespoon nut butters, ½ ounce (about 15) nuts, about 20 medium olives, ⅓ of an avocado.

Rationale: Sure, these foods are high in fat, but it's monounsaturated fat, the type that's actually necessary for good health.

Seventh tier (optional): No more than 4–5 servings a week each of skinless breast meat of poultry; eggs (you can actually have up to 7 servings a week); refined grains.

Serving size: 3 ounces of poultry, 1 egg, 1 slice of bread, ½ English muffin, ½ hamburger bun, ½ bagel, ½ cup of cooked cereal or pasta.

Rationale: Skinless breast meat is low in saturated fat and an excellent source of protein and iron. Whole eggs needn't be taboo: Research suggests that for nondiabetics, even eating an egg every day won't raise disease risk. Refined grains give you carbohydrates, but they've been stripped of most vitamins, minerals, and fiber, then various vitamins and nutrients are added back in. Whole grains are the better option.

Eighth tier (optional): No more than 4–5 servings a week of polyunsaturated fats such as salad dressing, mayonnaise, or vegetable oils (other than olive and canola).

Serving size: 1 tablespoon.

Rationale: Polyunsaturated fats don't raise heart disease risk, but they may increase risk of breast, colon, and pancreatic cancers. Small amounts don't seem to be harmful, however.

Ninth tier (optional): No more than 3–4 servings a month of red meat; or poultry other than breast meat.

Serving size: 3 ounces.

Rationale: Red meat is a rich source of iron and zinc, but it's loaded with artery-clogging saturated fat. Eating more than 12–16 ounces a month increases your risk of colon cancer and heart disease. Don't be fooled into thinking that chicken and turkey are necessarily healthier than red meat: Cuts other than breast meat are also high in saturated fat.

Tenth tier (optional): Limit or avoid saturated fats such as butter and fatty dairy products, trans fatty acids, and alcohol.

Rationale: Saturated fats and trans fatty acids have absolutely no nutritional value and are major culprits in the development of heart disease. Trans fats are created when polyunsaturated oils are turned from liquid to solids, and often used to keep baked goods fresh. While alcohol may help prevent heart disease, it also raises the risk of breast cancer. You may want to discuss your health risks with your physician.

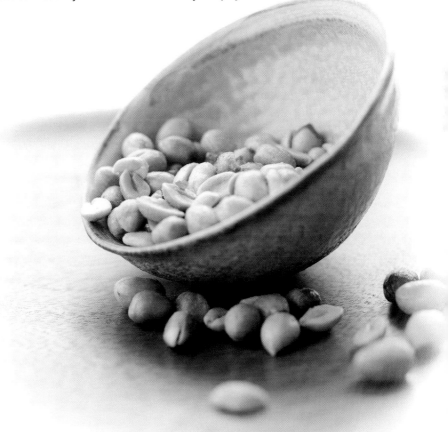

if you're a vegetarian (or vegan)

Research suggests that vegetarians enjoy a longer life expectancy than carnivores; and lower rates of heart disease, hypertension, type-II diabetes, and colorectal cancer. But only, of course, if you eat a healthy vegetarian diet—theoretically you could be a vegetarian and live on ice cream and cookies! Can you meet your daily nutrient requirements simply by removing meat or all animal products from the *Shape®* Pyramid? Yes, if you carefully select your foods and:

1. Take a vitamin supplement to ensure adequate intake of zinc, omega-3s, and vitamins B_{12} and B_6, which are naturally found abundantly only in animal products.

2. If you eliminate dairy products as well as meat, compensate for the calcium deficit by drinking orange juice or soy milk fortified with vitamin D and calcium and loading up on calcium-rich vegetables. A calcium supplement may also be in order. Avoiding meat means that you need to get your iron from legumes and fortified cereals. It's smart to consume your iron sources with vitamin C, which helps your body absorb plant-based iron. Getting enough protein may also require planning; a scoop of garbanzo beans isn't going to cut it. Eggs and low-fat dairy products can provide some. If you're a vegan, you'll want to turn to fortified soy products—tofu, soy milk, and/or edamame beans. Nuts and combo meals of whole grains and legumes also boost your protein intake.

3. If you're planning to get pregnant, consult with a dietitian who's experienced in the vegetarian or vegan lifestyles.

the Shape® pyramid meal plan

Here's a 4-week eating plan from our pyramid. It supplies everything you need. The daily calorie count is around 2,000. You can tweak this either way by about 200 calories. If you're very active (you do 45 minutes of cardio 4 times a week and strength-train twice a week) you'll need more. Get the calories mostly from additional fruits and vegetables, whole grains, legumes, and low-fat dairy products.

If you're on a weight-loss program, limit your intake to about 1,800 calories. Go below this amount and your metabolism may slow to a crawl, foiling your efforts to lose weight. It's important to get sufficient calories and spread them throughout the day. Undereating is a common trigger for bingeing later. Use egg substitutes or two egg whites for one whole egg, and fresh fruit for prepared desserts. Alternatively, step up your aerobic activity to burn an additional 200 calories a day.

week one

day one

Nutrition Score: 1,979 calories, 18% fat (40 g: 11 g saturated), 65% carbohydrates (322 g), 17% protein (84 g), 48 g fiber, 1,615 mg calcium, 17 mg iron, 2,254 mg sodium

Breakfast

Breakfast Focaccia with Smoked Salmon and Capers
Spread 2 tablespoons nonfat cream cheese on 1 slice whole-grain bread. Top with 1 tablespoon capers and 1 ounce smoked salmon.

1 cup blueberries

8 ounces nonfat milk

8 ounces water

Midmorning Snack

Zucchini with Curry Dip
1 sliced zucchini with a purée of ½ cup light silken tofu and 1 teaspoon curry powder.

½ cup dried apple slices

16 ounces water

Lunch

Creamy Asparagus Soup

Simmer 2 cups chopped asparagus in 2 cups water or reduced-sodium vegetable broth for 10 minutes. Purée in a blender with ¼ cup nonfat sour cream.

1 Garlic-Chive Roll

Defrost (½ pound) frozen whole-wheat bread dough (see package directions). Knead in 1 tablespoon minced chives and ¼ teaspoon garlic powder. Shape into 8 round rolls; bake on a baking sheet 15 minutes at 425°F. Freeze remaining 7 rolls up to two months.

1 banana

8 ounces water

Midafternoon Snack

Herbed Goat Cheese

Mix together 2 tablespoons soft goat cheese and 2 teaspoons chopped fresh herbs.

2 crisp rye crackers

4 Kalamata (Greek) olives

16 ounces water

Dinner

Linguine with Clam Sauce

Sauté 1 minced garlic clove in 1 teaspoon olive oil for 2 minutes. Add 1 drained 6-ounce can minced clams and sauté 2 minutes. Add a mixture of 1 tablespoon whole-wheat flour and 1 cup nonfat milk to clams. Simmer 2 minutes until thickened. Toss with 1½ cups cooked whole-wheat linguini and 2 tablespoons chopped parsley.

Baby Spinach Salad

Combine 2 teaspoons olive oil, 2 tablespoons red wine vinegar, ¼ teaspoon pepper, and ¼ cup diced mushrooms. Toss with 2 cups baby spinach leaves and 2 cherry tomatoes.

1 slice multigrain bread with seeds

8 ounces water

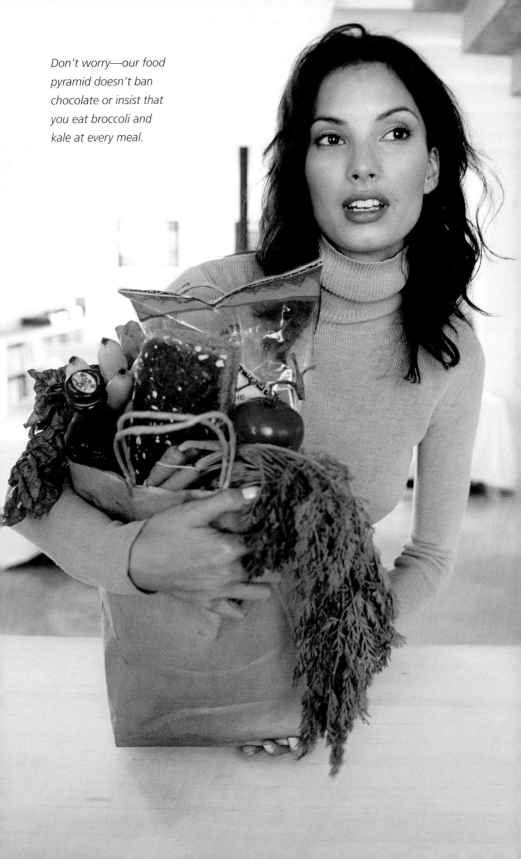

Don't worry—our food pyramid doesn't ban chocolate or insist that you eat broccoli and kale at every meal.

Dessert

Decaf Mocha Latte
Combine ½ cup decaffeinated coffee, ½ cup scalded nonfat milk, and 1 teaspoon each unsweetened cocoa and sugar.

2 biscotti cookies with nuts

½ cup nonfat berry sorbet

8 ounces water

day two

Nutrition Score: 1,987 calories, 20% fat (44 g: 7 g saturated), 62% carbohydrates (308 g), 18% protein (89 g), 43 g fiber, 1,523 mg calcium, 19 mg iron, 2,032 mg sodium

Breakfast

Smothered French Toast
Coat 2 slices whole-grain bread in a mixture of 1 egg and 1 tablespoon nonfat milk. Sauté in nonstick skillet 3 minutes a side. Top with ½ cup applesauce and 1 tablespoon chopped walnuts.

8 ounces orange juice

8 ounces water

Midmorning Snack

Tortilla Chips and Salsa
Cut 1 whole-wheat flour tortilla into wedges. Coat with olive oil spray; bake on a baking sheet at 350°F for 10 minutes. Sprinkle with ⅛ teaspoon salt. Serve with blend of 1 diced tomato and 2 tablespoon chopped cilantro and 1 tablespoon lime juice.

16 ounces water

Lunch

Quinoa Salad with Red Peppers and Pine Nuts
Toss together 1 cup cooked quinoa; 2 tablespoons diced, water-packed roasted red peppers; 2 tablespoons sherry vinegar; and 1 teaspoon olive oil. Toast 1 tablespoon pine nuts in hot nonstick skillet for 2 minutes. Spoon quinoa mixture onto 1 cup red lettuce leaves. Top with pine nuts.

1 peach

8 ounces water

Midafternoon Snack

Frozen Cinnamon Cappuccino
In a blender, purée ½ cup coffee, 1 cup nonfat milk, 4 ice cubes, and ¼ teaspoon cinnamon. Top with 2 tablespoons bran cereal.

16 ounces water

Dinner

Barbecued Roasted Chicken
Coat ½ skinless chicken breast (4 ounces) with 1 tablespoon lemon juice and ½ teaspoon each brown sugar, chili powder, and coriander. Roast in roasting pan for 25 minutes at 400°F.

Tarragon Mashed Potatoes
Boil 1 peeled and cubed potato in water for 10 minutes. Mash with ⅓ cup nonfat sour cream, 2 tablespoons minced fresh tarragon, and ½ teaspoon each salt and black pepper.

Wilted Greens with Sesame Seeds
Sauté 1 teaspoon sesame seeds in 2 teaspoons olive oil. Add 2 cups chopped kale; cover and steam 1 minute.

8 ounces water

Dessert

Bottomless Apple Tart
Combine 1 sliced apple and 1 tablespoon maple syrup in a baking dish; top with a mixture of 3 tablespoons oats, ¼ teaspoon nutmeg, and 2 teaspoons each whole-wheat flour and sliced almonds. Bake 30 minutes at 400°F. Serve with ½ cup nonfat vanilla yogurt.

8 ounces water

day three

Nutrition Score: 2,085 calories, 12% fat (28 g: 6 g saturated), 70% carbohydrates (365 g), 18% protein (94 g), 62 g fiber, 1,450 mg calcium, 26 mg iron, 1,703 mg sodium

Breakfast

Fresh Fruit Parfait
In a tall glass, layer 1 cup any flavor low-fat yogurt, 1 sliced kiwi, 1 cup blackberries, and 1 cup whole-grain or bran cereal.

1 slice whole-grain toast with 1 teaspoon apple butter

8 ounces water

Midmorning Snack

Three-Bean Salad with Cilantro
Combine ¼ cup each canned and drained pink, black, and white beans with 1 tablespoon each rice wine vinegar (or mirin) and chopped fresh cilantro.

1 orange

16 ounces water

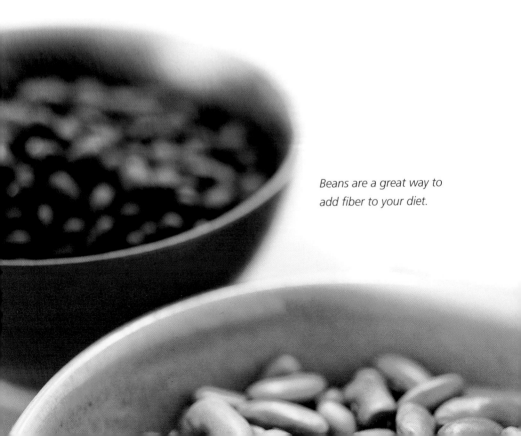

Beans are a great way to add fiber to your diet.

Lunch

Grilled Tuna Salad with Couscous and Mustard Greens
Season both sides of a 4-ounce tuna steak with black pepper.
Grill or broil 3 minutes per side. Pull apart with a fork and toss
with ¼ cup diced, oil-packed artichoke hearts; 1 cup each red
bell pepper and snap peas; and 1 tablespoon red wine vinegar.
Spoon ½ cup cooked whole-wheat couscous onto 2 cups mustard green leaves. Top with tuna mixture.

2 whole-grain crackers

1 nectarine

8 ounces water

Midafternoon Snack

Oven-Roasted Chestnuts
Slice small X's on the ends of 5 chestnuts. Roast in roasting pan
for 30 minutes at 400°F.

4 ounces nonfat milk

1 tangerine

16 ounces water

Dinner

Spinach Fettuccini with Sun-Dried Tomato Sauce
In a blender, purée 1 cup water or vegetable broth, 1 tomato,
2 tablespoons dry-packed sun-dried tomatoes, 2 tablespoons
balsamic vinegar, and ¼ teaspoon black pepper. Pour over 1 cup
cooked spinach fettuccini.

2 cups mixed greens with 1 tablespoon nonfat dressing

1 mixed-grain roll

8 ounces water

Dessert

Angel Food Napoleon
Halve 1 slice angel food cake horizontally. Spread ¼ cup low-fat
strawberry yogurt on bottom half. Top with ¼ cup sliced strawberries. Top with second cake slice, ¼ cup low-fat strawberry
yogurt, and ¼ cup sliced strawberries.

8 ounces water

day four

Nutrition Score: 2,043 calories, 24% fat (54 g: 15 g saturated), 57% carbohydrates (291 g), 19% protein (97 g), 49 g fiber, 1,241 mg calcium, 25 mg iron, 1,909 mg sodium

Breakfast

Egg Strata with Spinach and Feta Cheese
Combine 3 egg whites, 1 cup chopped spinach, 1 slice cubed whole-grain bread, and 1 tablespoon crumbled feta cheese. Cook in 2 teaspoons olive oil in an oven-proof skillet for 3 minutes until egg whites are set. Then broil until surface is cooked.

1 cup pineapple chunks

8 ounces nonfat milk

8 ounces water

Midmorning Snack

Papaya Swirl
Mix together ⅓ cup part-skim ricotta cheese and 1 cup diced papaya. Top with ¼ cup whole-grain cereal or 2 tablespoons toasted flaxseeds

16 ounces water

Lunch

Lentil Salad with Pasta and Green Peas
Toss together 1 cup each cooked whole-wheat pasta and ¼ cup cooked lentils, 1 cup green peas, 2 teaspoons olive oil, and 2 tablespoons each minced red onion and white wine vinegar. Serve over 1 cup romaine lettuce.

1 plum

8 ounces water

Midafternoon Snack

Corn Chips with White Bean Dip
Mash together until smooth ⅓ cup canned, drained white beans, and ¼ teaspoon each ground cumin and onion powder. Serve with 1 ounce baked corn chips.

1 apple

16 ounces water

Dinner

Jamaican Jerk Chicken

Mix together 1 tablespoon cider vinegar; ½ teaspoon each allspice, cloves, basil, and thyme; and ¼ teaspoon each salt and black pepper. Rub all over ½ skinless chicken breast (4 ounces). Cook in roasting pan 25 minutes at 400°F.

Green Beans with Wild Mushrooms

Sauté 1 cup sliced shiitake (or regular button) mushrooms in 2 teaspoons olive oil for 3 minutes. Add 1 cup trimmed green beans; sauté 3 minutes. Season with ¼ teaspoon each salt and black pepper.

Rosemary Roasted Sweet Potato

Quick Tip: *Nuts are among the most nutritious foods you can consume, containing vitamin E and heart-healthy monounsaturated fats. Plus, research shows that eating a few nuts (about a small handful) on a regular basis can keep you on your healthful eating plan by helping you feel full longer.*

Cube 1 sweet potato; toss with 2 teaspoons olive oil and 1 teaspoon chopped fresh rosemary. Transfer to a baking sheet and roast 35 minutes at 400°F.

8 ounces water

Dessert

Thai Pudding

Mix together ½ cup vanilla pudding made with nonfat milk. Toast 1 tablespoon coconut on a baking sheet for 5 minutes at 350°F. Sprinkle it and ⅛ teaspoon ground ginger over pudding.

1 cup cubed mango

8 ounces water

day five

Nutrition Score: 2,020 calories, 22% fat (49 g: 14 g saturated), 60% carbohydrates (303 g), 18% protein (91 g), 47 g fiber, 1,598 mg calcium, 18 mg iron, 2,034 mg sodium

Breakfast

¾ cup low-fat granola with 1 tablespoon minced dried apricots

1 cup light vanilla-flavored, calcium- and vitamin D-fortified soy milk

½ grapefruit

8 ounces water

Midmorning Snack

1 whole-wheat pita

2 tablespoons hummus

1 cup grapes

16 ounces water

Lunch

Whole-Grain Bread Salad with
Tomatoes and Mozzarella

Bake 2 slices whole-grain bread on a baking sheet for 5 minutes at 350°F. Cut into small cubes. In a large bowl, soak cubes in 2 cups warm water 5 minutes.

Drain, squeeze out water. Add 1 diced tomato, 1 teaspoon olive oil, 2 tablespoons each chopped fresh basil and balsamic vinegar, and 1 ounce diced part-skim mozzarella cheese.

1 cup cubed cantaloupe

8 ounces water

Midafternoon Snack

Fruit Fondue

Combine ⅓ cup part-skim ricotta cheese and ¼ teaspoon almond extract. Serve with 1 Granny Smith apple, sliced.

16 ounces water

Dinner

Parmesan-Crusted Bluefish

Mix together 2 teaspoons grated Parmesan cheese, ½ teaspoon dried rosemary, ¼ teaspoon black pepper, and 1 tablespoon each whole-grain bread crumbs and lemon juice. Press mixture into sides of a 4-ounce bluefish fillet (or mackerel or trout). Cook in roasting pan for 15–20 minutes at 400°F.

Brown Rice Pilaf with Toasted Pumpkin Seeds

Sauté 2 tablespoons pumpkin seeds in 1 teaspoon olive oil for 3 minutes. Add ¼ cup uncooked brown rice and ½ teaspoon dried oregano; sauté 1 minute. Add ⅔ cup water or vegetable broth. Simmer 30 minutes until liquid is absorbed. Add ¼ teaspoon each salt and pepper.

2 cups steamed broccoli with 1 tablespoon fresh lemon juice

8 ounces nonfat milk

8 ounces water

Dessert

Poached Pear with Raspberry Coulis

Peel, halve, and core 1 pear. Microwave 5 minutes in shallow dish covered with plastic. Simmer 1 cup raspberries with 1 teaspoon confectioners' sugar for 5 minutes. Strain. Pour sauce over pear.

8 ounces water

Mistake to Avoid:

The United States Department of Agriculture (USDA) Food Guide Pyramid doesn't distinguish between full-fat, low-fat, and nonfat dairy products—but you should! The fat in whole milk and whole-milk cheeses is the same heart-damaging saturated fat that's found in red meat.

day six

Nutrition Score: 2,045 calories, 19% fat (43 g: 9 g saturated), 64% carbohydrates (327 g), 17% protein (87 g), 62 g fiber, 1,066 mg calcium, 18 mg iron, 1,651 mg sodium

Breakfast

Oats with Apple and Cranberries
In a microwave-safe bowl, combine ½ cup calcium-fortified soy milk, ⅓ cup oats, 1 diced apple, 1 tablespoon dried cranberries, and ½ teaspoon cinnamon. Cover with plastic wrap and microwave on high 2–3 minutes until liquid is absorbed.

4 ounces grapefruit juice

8 ounces water

Midmorning Snack

Tropical Trail Mix
Combine ¼ cup Grape Nuts cereal and 1 tablespoon each slivered almonds and dried papaya.

1 orange

8 ounces water

Lunch

Spicy Sesame Noodles with Carrots, Broccoli, and Peanuts
Cook 2 ounces soba (buckwheat) noodles according to package directions. Drain and toss with 1 cup fresh broccoli florets, ¼ cup shredded carrots, and 1 teaspoon each reduced-sodium soy sauce and sesame oil. Serve over 2 Romaine lettuce leaves. Top with 1 tablespoon dry roasted peanuts.

1 cup blackberries

8 ounces water

Midafternoon Snack

Peanut Butter-Banana Wrap
Top 1 whole-wheat tortilla with 1 tablespoon reduced-fat peanut butter and 1 banana. Roll up.

2 kiwis

8 ounces water

Dinner

Garlic-Drenched Chicken
Season ½ skinless, boneless chicken breast (4 ounces) with salt, black pepper, and ½ teaspoon onion powder. Rub chicken all over with 2 minced garlic cloves. Roast at 400°F for 25 minutes until cooked through.

Cumin-Dusted Red Potatoes
Quarter 2 small red potatoes. Toss potatoes with 2 teaspoons olive oil and 1 teaspoon ground cumin. Roast at 400°F for 35 minutes until tender and golden.

Portobello Mushrooms with Spinach and Smoked Mozzarella
Top 1 portobello mushroom cap (stem removed) with 1 cup fresh spinach leaves and 1 ounce smoked mozzarella cheese. Bake at 400°F for 10 minutes until cheese melts.

8 ounces water

Dessert

Chocolate-Raspberry Milkshake
Combine in a blender: ½ cup fat-free vanilla frozen yogurt, ½ cup nonfat milk, 1 cup frozen raspberries, and 1 tablespoon chocolate syrup. Puree until smooth.

day seven

Nutrition Score: 2,034 calories, 18% fat (41 g: 7 g saturated), 65% carbohydrates (331 g), 17% protein (86 g), 50 g fiber, 1,019 mg calcium, 16 mg iron, 1,963 mg sodium

Breakfast

Egg White Omelette with Roasted Red Peppers and Basil
Spray a large nonstick skillet with cooking spray. Set pan over medium-high heat and add 3 egg whites. Cook until egg is cooked through to the surface. Top 1 half with ½ cup thinly sliced roasted red peppers (from water-packed jar) and 2 tablespoons chopped fresh basil. Fold over and cook 1 minute to heat through. Season to taste with salt and black pepper.

1 cup cubed cantaloupe

4 ounces calcium-fortified orange juice

8 ounces water

Midmorning Snack

¼ cup roasted soy nuts

1 cup seedless grapes

8 ounces water

Lunch

Gazpacho-Shrimp Salad with Couscous

Bring ¾ cup water to a boil. Add ½ cup whole-wheat couscous, cover and remove from heat. Let stand 5 minutes. Meanwhile, in a medium saucepan over medium-high heat, combine 4 ounces peeled and deveined shrimp and enough water to cover. Bring to a boil. Once water boils and shrimp are bright pink, drain and plunge shrimp into ice water to prevent further cooking. In a large bowl, combine 1 cup canned diced tomatoes, ⅓ cup diced cucumber, ½ diced yellow bell pepper, and 1 tablespoon chopped fresh basil. Add shrimp and toss to combine. Season to taste with salt and black pepper. Serve shrimp mixture over couscous.

1 pear

8 ounces water

Midafternoon Snack

¼ cup walnuts with ¼ cup dried cherries

1 starfruit (carambola)

8 ounces water

Dinner

Curried Pumpkin Soup with Potatoes

Heat 2 teaspoons olive oil in a large saucepan over medium-high heat. Add ¼ cup diced onion and sauté 2 minutes. Add 1 teaspoon curry powder and ¼ teaspoon ground black pepper and stir to coat. Add 1½ cups reduced-sodium chicken broth, 1 cup canned pumpkin, and 1 peeled, cubed potato. Bring to a boil. Reduce heat to medium, partially cover and simmer 8–10 minutes until potatoes are tender. Remove from heat and stir in 1 tablespoon chopped fresh cilantro.

Creamy Red Cabbage Slaw

Combine 1 cup shredded red cabbage, 2 tablespoons fat-free mayonnaise, and 1 tablespoon fresh lemon juice. Mix to coat cabbage. Season to taste with salt and black pepper.

1 whole-grain roll (2 ounces)

8 ounces water

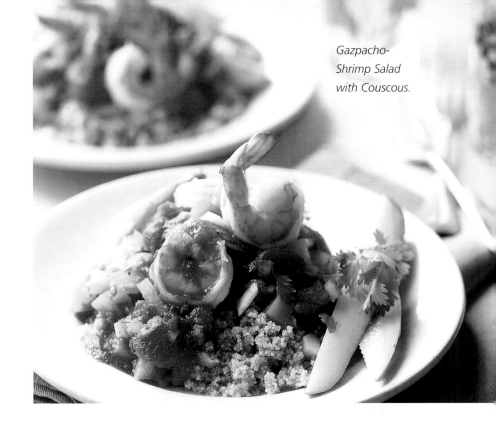

*Gazpacho-
Shrimp Salad
with Couscous.*

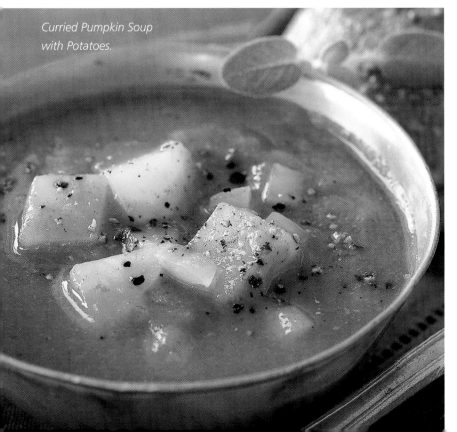

*Curried Pumpkin Soup
with Potatoes.*

Dessert

Caramelized Grapefruit with Vanilla Yogurt
Top ½ grapefruit with 1 teaspoon light brown sugar. Place
under broiler and cook 1–2 minutes, until golden brown. Serve
with ½ cup low-fat vanilla yogurt.

week two

day one

Nutrition Score: 1,962 calories, 15% fat (33 g: 7 g saturated), 68% carbohydrates
(334 g), 17% protein (83 g), 39 g fiber, 1,114 mg calcium, 27 mg iron, 1,193 mg sodium

Breakfast

Banana-Soy Shake
Combine in a blender: 1 banana, ½ cup calcium-fortified vanilla
soy milk, and ½ cup calcium-fortified orange juice. Puree until
smooth.

2 slices whole-grain toast with 2 teaspoons trans fat-free light
margarine

8 ounces water

Midmorning Snack

1 low-fat cinnamon-raisin granola bar

1 pear

8 ounces water

Lunch

Smoked Trout on Pumpernickel with Cucumber
Whisk together 1 tablespoon fat-free mayonnaise and 1 teaspoon each chopped fresh dill and fresh lemon juice. Spread
mixture on 1 slice of pumpernickel bread. Top with 3 ounces
smoked trout (or smoked salmon) and ¼ cup thinly sliced
cucumber. Top with second slice of bread.

1 sliced beefsteak tomato drizzled with 1 teaspoon balsamic
vinegar

2 blood oranges or 1 regular orange

8 ounces water

Midafternoon Snack

1 cup strawberry or peach sorbet with 1 cup fresh strawberries

8 ounces water

Dinner

Spaghetti Bolognese
Cook 4 ounces ground turkey breast in a hot, nonstick skillet until browned. Add 1 cup reduced-sodium tomato sauce, 1 tablespoon chopped fresh basil, ½ teaspoon dried oregano, and ¼ teaspoon ground black pepper. Simmer 5 minutes. Spoon sauce over 2 ounces cooked whole-wheat pasta, and top with 1 tablespoon grated Parmesan cheese.

1 cup each sliced zucchini and yellow squash (serve raw or microwave on high 2 minutes). Season to taste with salt and black pepper.

8 ounces water

Dessert

6 amaretti cookies with ½ cup low-fat cookie dough ice cream

2 cups cubed watermelon (or any melon variety)

day two

Nutrition Score: 2,047 calories, 21% fat (48 g: 11 g saturated), 63% carbohydrates (322 g), 16% protein (82 g), 45 g fiber, 1,115 mg calcium, 21 mg iron, 2,440 mg sodium

Breakfast

Heart-Smart Breakfast Sandwich
Spray a nonstick skillet with cooking spray and place over medium-high heat. Add 1 egg and cook 2 minutes per side, until yolk is cooked. Toast 1 oat bran English muffin. Top ½ muffin with 1 ounce soy cheese. Top with cooked egg and second muffin half.

4 ounces sugar-free cranberry juice

8 ounces water

Midmorning Snack

1 fat-free oatmeal raisin cookie

1 cup cubed papaya

8 ounces water

Lunch

Salmon Salad
Combine one 3-ounce can water-packed salmon (drained),
¼ cup minced red onion, 1 tablespoon fat-free mayonnaise,
1 teaspoon drained capers, and ½ teaspoon Dijon mustard.
Mix well and spoon over 2 cups baby spinach leaves.

2 slices whole-grain rye bread topped with 2 teaspoons fat-free
cream cheese

2 plums

8 ounces water

Midafternoon Snack

1 cup low-sodium split pea soup with 4 sesame bread sticks
(Barbara's Bakery)

1 cup green grapes

8 ounces water

Dinner

Sweet Pea and Onion Risotto
Heat 2 teaspoons olive oil in a large saucepan over medium
heat. Add ½ cup Arborio (short grain) rice and 2 minced garlic
cloves. Cook 2 minutes until rice is golden, stirring frequently.
Add ½ cup reduced-sodium chicken broth and simmer until liquid is absorbed, stirring frequently. Add another cup of broth,
½ cup at a time, waiting until liquid is absorbed before adding
the next ½ cup (total cooking time is about 20 minutes). Stir in
1 cup pearl onions and ½ cup frozen green peas, and cook 2
minutes. Remove from heat and season to taste with salt and
black pepper.

Sundried Tomato Crostini
Top 1 slice toasted sourdough bread with 1 teaspoon prepared
sundried tomato pesto.

2 cups steamed broccoli

8 ounces water

Dessert

½ cup chocolate sorbet with 1 cup raspberries (fresh or frozen)

day three

Nutrition Score: 2,011 calories, 16% fat (36 g: 7 g saturated), 70% carbohydrates (352 g), 14% protein (70 g), 33 g fiber, 1,181 mg calcium, 10 mg iron, 2,461 mg sodium

Breakfast

1 whole-grain waffle (Eggo) with 1 tablespoon maple syrup

½ grapefruit

8 ounces calcium-fortified cranberry juice

8 ounces water

Midmorning Snack

2 hard pretzels with 1 tablespoon honey mustard
10 baby carrots
8 ounces water

Lunch

Japanese Noodle Salad

Heat 2 teaspoons sesame oil in a large nonstick skillet over medium-high heat. Add 1 minced garlic clove and 2 teaspoons chopped fresh ginger, and sauté 1 minute. Add 2 cups frozen sugar snap stir-fry mix (Bird's Eye) and sauté 2 minutes, until vegetables are crisp-tender. Add vegetable mixture to 2 ounces cooked udon (brown rice) noodles or whole-wheat spaghetti, and toss to combine. Top with 1 tablespoon roasted soy nuts before serving.

8 ounces water

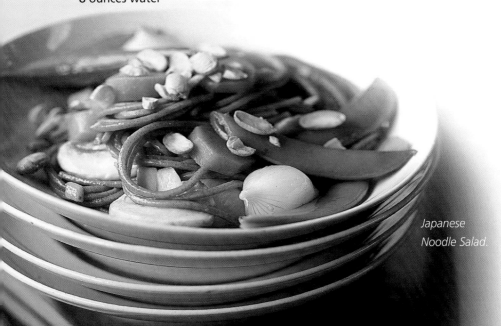

Japanese Noodle Salad.

Midafternoon Snack

1 cup low-fat vanilla yogurt mixed with ¼ cup mandarin oranges (in light syrup)

1 cup sliced zucchini with 2 tablespoons fat-free ranch dressing

8 ounces water

Dinner

Chicken with Apple, Baby Onions, and Sweet Potato

Heat 2 teaspoons olive oil in a large saucepan over medium-high heat. Season ½ skinless, boneless chicken breast (4 ounces) with salt and black pepper and add to pan. Sauté 2 minutes per side until golden brown. Add 1 cup reduced-sodium chicken broth, ½ cup frozen small white onions, 1 peeled and cubed sweet potato, 1 cubed apple, and ½ teaspoon dried thyme, and bring to a simmer. Cook 8 minutes, until potatoes are tender and chicken is cooked through.

½ cup cooked instant brown rice

1 cup steamed Italian or French green beans

8 ounces water

Dessert

2-ounce slice angel food cake with 1 cup sliced peaches and 2 tablespoons caramel topping

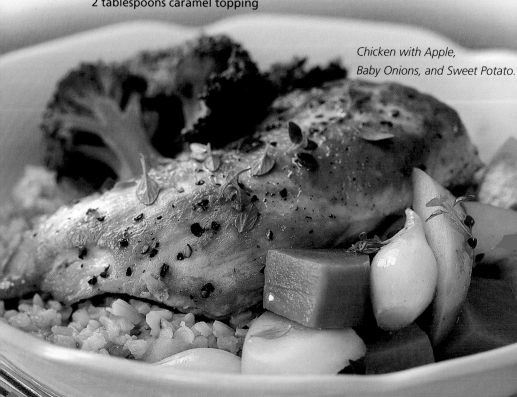

Chicken with Apple, Baby Onions, and Sweet Potato.

day four

Nutrition Score: 2,036 calories, 14% fat (32 g: 11 g saturated), 69% carbohydrates (351 g), 17% protein (87 g), 48 g fiber, 1,335 mg calcium, 12 mg iron, 2,527 mg sodium

Breakfast

Indian Tofu Scramble
Combine in a bowl: 3 ounces diced firm tofu, ¼ cup diced tomatoes (fresh or canned), ½ teaspoon each curry powder and ground cumin, and 2 teaspoons chopped fresh cilantro. Sauté mixture in a hot skillet for 5 minutes, stirring frequently until mixture thickens.

2 slices whole-wheat toast with 2 teaspoons fruit preserves

8 ounces grapefruit juice

8 ounces water

Midmorning Snack

Creamy Fruit Salad
Combine 1 cup each cubed honeydew melon, orange wedges, and red grapes; 1 cup low-fat vanilla yogurt (dairy or soy); and 1 teaspoon chopped fresh mint. Toss.

8 ounces water

Lunch

Warm Lentil Salad
Combine in a bowl: one 19-ounce can Progresso 99% Fat-Free Lentil Soup and ½ cup uncooked instant brown rice. Cover with plastic wrap and microwave on high 5 minutes. Let stand 5 minutes. Add ¼ cup each, diced carrots, and yellow or green bell pepper, and 1 tablespoon red wine vinegar. Toss with a fork to combine. Serve over 2 red lettuce leaves.

1 cup cubed watermelon

8 ounces water

Midafternoon Snack

1 reduced-calorie ice cream sandwich (Weight Watchers)

1 cup cherry tomatoes

8 ounces water

Dinner

Tomato-Vegetable Puree with Lump Crabmeat
Combine in a blender or food processor: 2 chopped tomatoes, ½ cup low-sodium tomato juice, ½ green bell pepper, ⅓ cup sliced cucumber, 2 teaspoons fresh lemon juice, and ¼ teaspoon black pepper. Puree until almost smooth, leaving some larger pieces. Pour mixture into a shallow bowl and top with ½ cup fresh or canned (6-ounce can) lump crabmeat.

1 whole-grain roll (2 ounces) with 2 teaspoons trans fat-free light margarine

2 cups mixed lettuce greens topped with 2 tablespoons each crumbled feta cheese and fat-free Catalina dressing

8 ounces water

Dessert

4 reduced-fat chocolate chip cookies (Healthy Choice)

1 cup cherries (fresh or frozen)

day five

Nutrition Score: 2,050 calories, 16% fat (36 g: 9 g saturated), 63% carbohydrates (323 g), 21% protein (108 g), 59 g fiber, 1,145 mg calcium, 13 mg iron, 2,243 mg sodium

Breakfast

Mixed Berry Smoothie
Combine in a blender: 1 cup each frozen raspberries and blackberries, 1 cup low-fat strawberry yogurt, and 1 teaspoon wheat germ. Puree until smooth.

1 slice whole-grain bread with 1 teaspoon trans fat-free light margarine

8 ounces water

Midmorning Snack

2 honey graham crackers with 1 tablespoon reduced-fat peanut butter

1 apple

8 ounces water

Lunch

Fajita-Beef Salad

Place 1 whole-wheat four tortilla on a baking sheet and sprinkle with ½ teaspoon cumin. Bake at 400°F for 8 minutes until golden. Remove from oven, transfer to a plate. Set aside. In a large skillet, combine 1 tablespoon reduced-sodium soy sauce, ½ teaspoon liquid smoke, and ¼ teaspoon ground cumin. Set pan over medium-high heat and bring mixture to a simmer. Add 2 cups frozen pepper stir-fry mix (Bird's Eye) and cook 3 minutes, until tender. Add 3 ounces sliced lean roast beef and cook 2 minutes until hot. Top toasted tortilla with ¼ cup shredded lettuce, and then top with roast beef mixture.

8 ounces water

Midafternoon Snack

5 Greek olives (Kalamata) with 4 rye crispbread crackers

1 sliced tomato

8 ounces water

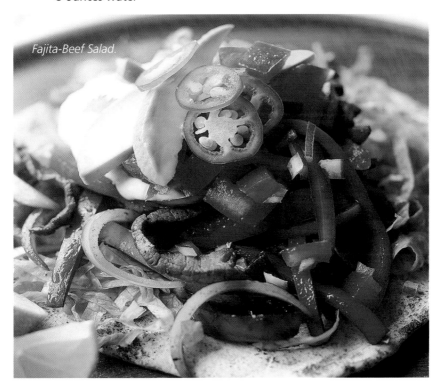

Fajita-Beef Salad.

Dinner

Chicken Satay with Rice and Peas

Set a large nonstick skillet over medium-high heat. Add ½ skin-less, boneless chicken breast (4 ounces), and sauté 2–3 minutes until golden brown on both sides. Season with salt and black pepper and remove from heat. Slice into thin strips. Mean-while, in a small saucepan, combine ⅓ cup reduced-sodium chicken broth, 1 tablespoon reduced-fat peanut butter, and 2 teaspoons reduced-sodium soy sauce. Simmer 2 minutes until hot, stirring frequently with a wire whisk. Serve chicken strips with peanut sauce on the side.

½ cup cooked brown rice mixed with 1 cup green peas and 1 chopped green onion

8 ounces water

Dessert

Mango with Ginger Cream

Whisk together 1 cup low-fat vanilla yogurt and ¼ teaspoon ground ginger. Serve with 1 sliced mango.

day six

Nutrition Score: 2,001 calories, 22% fat (49 g: 11 g saturated), 57% carbohydrates (285 g), 21% protein (105 g), 48 g fiber, 1,289 mg calcium, 17 mg iron, 1,801 mg sodium

Breakfast

Spinach and Egg White Omelette

Heat 2 teaspoons olive oil in a small nonstick skillet over medium-high heat. Add 3 egg whites to hot pan and cook until almost cooked through to the surface, frequently lifting the sides to allow uncooked egg to slide underneath. Top one side with 1 cup fresh spinach leaves and 2 tablespoons minced red onion. Fold over untopped side and cook 1 minute until spinach wilts. Season to taste with salt and black pepper.

1 toasted whole-wheat English muffin with 2 teaspoons fruit preserves

1 cup fresh blueberries

8 ounces water

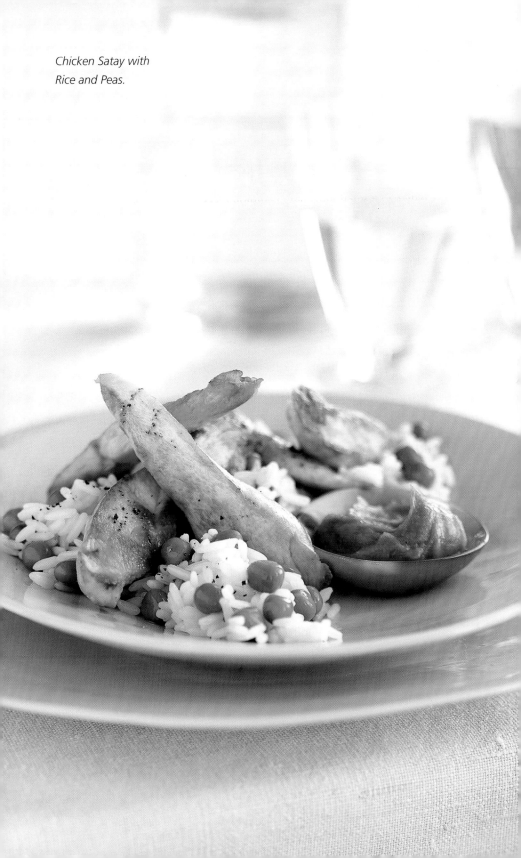

*Chicken Satay with
Rice and Peas.*

danger zones

There you are, full of good intentions and working at sticking to your healthy eating plan, when you run into all-too-familiar circumstances that really test your mettle. Here are four red-flag situations and how to deal with them.

1.   *A stress attack.* Food is a drug that alters brain chemistry and has a calming effect. That's why you may reach toward food when you're stressed and anxious. If you feel that you're about to run amok, ask yourself: "How much cookie dough ice cream do I really need to resolve the stress? One spoonful? Five? The entire half-gallon?" Obviously, the answer is that no amount will solve the problem, and overindulging will only compound your stress. Instead, face the stressful feelings. Write them down in your journal, take a bath, rent an uplifting movie, or take your dog for a walk. (You'll find more ideas for de-stressing in future chapters.)

2.   *A party.* Feeling festive, enjoying friends' company, and drinking alcohol can all cause you to lose your inhibitions at parties. But you won't feel remorseful the next day if you employ a few smart strategies. Hold your drink in your dominant hand. By relying on your "weak" hand to reach for eats, you cut back via a lack of coordination. Except for raw veggies and boiled shrimp, skip finger foods. This eliminates high-fat offerings such as chicken wings and cheese puffs. Survey the buffet table and decide what to eat before you load up; once it's on your plate, you'll likely eat it. Sip on bubbly water between each boozy libation to cut down on calories and keep a clear head. And concentrate on enjoying the company rather than the cuisine.

3.   *A fast-food joint.* Fast-food restaurants are a fact of modern life. They're ubiquitous and convenient for a rushed lunch. Most chains offer at least one or two low-fat options so you really can eat in a healthy way by making smart choices. Arm yourself with the nutritional skinny on fast-food menu items so you know going in what to order. Nearly all chains have Websites now, which give the nutritional breakdowns of their food. For instance, by going to **www.pizzahut.com**, you'll discover that there's a substantial difference in fat grams between a slice of chicken pizza and one with Italian sausage. If the fast-food outlet of your choice doesn't have a Website, ask the restaurant for the nutritional breakdown. Then if you really can't resist those french fries, occasionally factor them into your day's calorie budget, and compensate at other meals.

4.   *A routine.* Sometimes you feel like being in a rut, sometimes you don't. That daily bowl of high-fiber cereal, skim milk, and fruit is a fine breakfast and doesn't require a lot of thought and effort. Then one day you look at it and . . . *blah.* So you skip breakfast and end up raiding the vending machine at work. Keeping your healthy diet varied is the key to keeping it going. Yield to the allure of the unusual. Instead of automatically reaching for apples or broccoli, try one item you've never eaten before on each trip to the market. Instead of pasta, try soba, a nutty Japanese noodle made from buckwheat. You get the picture.

Midmorning Snack

1 apple with ¼ cup almonds

8 ounces water

Lunch

Grilled Chicken Salad

Top 2 cups chopped Romaine lettuce with ½ cup each chopped red bell pepper and sliced seedless cucumber, ¼ cup shredded carrot, and 2 tablespoons each crumbled feta cheese and chopped walnuts. Top with ½ grilled chicken breast (3 ounces) and 2 tablespoons fat-free Italian dressing.

5 reduced-fat whole-grain crackers

2 kiwis

8 ounces water

Midafternoon Snack

2 slices sprouted wheat or whole-grain bread with 2 tablespoons apple butter

8 ounces calcium-fortified orange juice or nonfat milk

8 ounces water

Dinner

Herb-Crusted Snapper

Preheat broiler. Season one 5-ounce snapper fillet with salt and black pepper. Rub 2 teaspoons each chopped fresh thyme and rosemary into fillet. Broil 3–5 minutes per side until fish is fork-tender.

2 cups chopped broccoli rabe, sautéed with 1 minced garlic clove in 2 teaspoons olive oil for 2–3 minutes until crisp-tender

½ cup cooked quick-cooking barley

8 ounces water

Dessert

Poached Pear with Raspberry Sauce

Halve and core 1 pear and place cut side up in a microwave-safe dish. Cover with plastic wrap and microwave on high 2 minutes until fork-tender. Top with 2 tablespoons of warmed raspberry preserves.

day seven

Nutrition Score: 1,977 calories, 23% fat (51 g: 14 g saturated), 63% carbohydrates (311 g), 14% protein (69 g), 39 g fiber, 989 mg calcium, 13 mg iron, 2,559 mg sodium

Breakfast

Maple-Almond Oats

Combine in a microwave-safe bowl: 1 cup nonfat milk, ½ cup rolled oats, and 1 tablespoon each slivered almonds and maple syrup. Cover with plastic wrap and microwave on high 2–3 minutes until liquid is absorbed.

½ grapefruit

8 ounces water

Midmorning Snack

1 banana with 1 tablespoon reduced-fat peanut butter

8 ounces water

Lunch

Turkey Wrap

Top one 8-inch whole-wheat tortilla with 2 teaspoons honey mustard. Top with 2 ounces turkey breast, 1 ounce reduced-fat Swiss cheese, ¼ cup watercress leaves, and 4 tomato slices. Sprinkle with ¼ teaspoon dried oregano and roll up.

1 orange

8 ounces water

Midafternoon Snack

½ whole-wheat pita with 1 teaspoon prepared basil pesto

2 cups cubed honeydew melon

8 ounces water

Dinner

Asian Noodles with Snow Peas,
Baby Carrots, and Cashews

Heat 2 teaspoons peanut oil in a large skillet over medium-high heat. Add 1 minced garlic clove and 1 teaspoon minced fresh ginger and cook 1 minute. Add 1 cup snow peas, 5 baby carrots, and 1 chopped green onion and cook 2 minutes. Spoon mixture over 2 ounces cooked soba (buckwheat) noodles and add 1 teaspoon sesame oil. Toss to combine. Top with 1 tablespoon chopped cashews.

Greek Salad

Top 2 cups of mixed greens (any combination of Romaine, Boston, and red lettuce) with ¼ cup sliced cucumber, 4 cherry tomatoes, and 2 teaspoons crumbled feta cheese. Top with 1 tablespoon fat-free Caesar or Italian dressing.

8 ounces water

Dessert

1 cup orange sherbet with 1 biscotti cookie

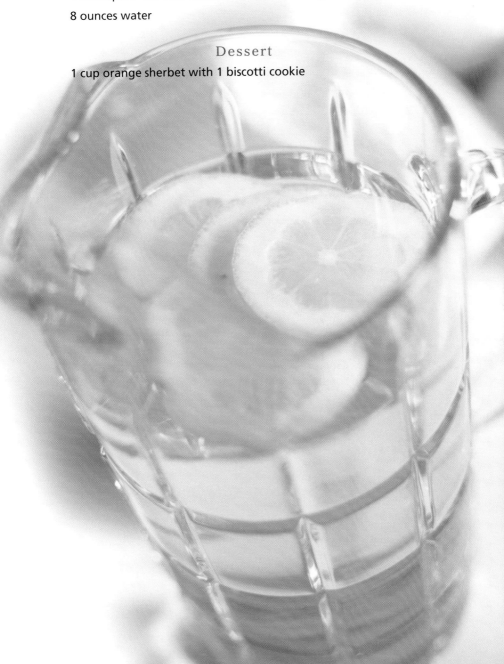

week three

day one

Nutrition Score: 2,037 calories, 23% fat (52 g: 8 g saturated), 59% carbohydrates (300 g), 18% protein (92 g), 50 g fiber, 1,039 mg calcium, 20 mg iron, 1,503 mg sodium

Breakfast

1 cup Raisin Bran cereal with ¾ cup calcium-fortified soy milk

Orange-Banana-Raspberry Smoothie
Combine in a blender: ½ cup calcium-fortified orange juice, 1 banana, and 1 cup frozen raspberries. Puree until smooth.

8 ounces water

Midmorning Snack

6-ounce container soy yogurt (any flavor) topped with 1 tablespoon peanuts

8 ounces water

Lunch

Tuna Salad with Wasabi Mayonnaise
Combine in a bowl: one 3-ounce can white water-packed tuna (drained), 2 tablespoons diced celery, 1 tablespoon fat-free mayonnaise, 1 teaspoon pickle relish, and ½ teaspoon wasabi paste. Mix to combine. Spoon mixture over 2 cups Boston or Bibb lettuce leaves.

1 slice whole-grain bread with 2 teaspoons fruit preserves

2 cups cubed pineapple

8 ounces water

Midafternoon Snack

2 cups air-popped popcorn mixed with ¼ cup slivered almonds

1 cup mandarin oranges (packed in light syrup, drained)

8 ounces water

Dinner

Pesto-Crusted Chicken

Coat ½ skinless, boneless chicken breast (4 ounces) with 2 tablespoons prepared basil pesto. Transfer chicken to a baking sheet that has been coated with cooking spray. Bake at 400°F for 25 minutes until cooked through.

1 baked sweet potato with 2 teaspoons trans fat-free light margarine

2 cups steamed broccoli

8 ounces water

Dessert

1 frozen fruit bar with 2 graham crackers

day two

Nutrition Score: 2,001 calories, 28% fat (62 g: 14 g saturated), 54% carbohydrates (270 g), 18% protein (90 g), 44 g fiber, 1,087 mg calcium, 11 mg iron, 2,177 mg sodium

Breakfast

1 whole-grain waffle (Eggo) with 1 cup strawberries (fresh or frozen) and 1 tablespoon maple syrup

Almond Latte

Combine ¾ cup brewed coffee, ¼ cup nonfat milk, and ¼ teaspoon almond extract.

8 ounces water

Midmorning Snack

1 cup dried apple slices with ¼ cup walnuts

8 ounces water

Quick Tip: *Get to know legumes, the family name for lentils, peas, all beans, and peanuts. They're high in protein while virtually free of saturated fats. A great source of soluble fiber to help you feel full and to aid digestion, legumes also contain valuable nutrients such as iron, potassium, folic acid (vitamin B₉), and cancer-fighting phytochemicals like isoflavones. And remember, canned beans are just as nutritious as dried— just give them a quick rinse to remove excess salt.*

Lunch

Bruschetta with Tomato, Mozzarella, and Basil
Halve one 2-ounce whole-wheat baguette lengthwise, and
brush both sides with 1 teaspoon olive oil. Set halves under the
broiler to toast. Top each toasted half with 2 tomato slices,
4 fresh basil leaves, and 1 ounce part-skim mozzarella cheese.

1 cup prepared lentil soup (Progresso)

1 banana

8 ounces water

Midafternoon Snack

1 cup cauliflower florets with 1 tablespoon fat-free ranch dressing

8 ounces water

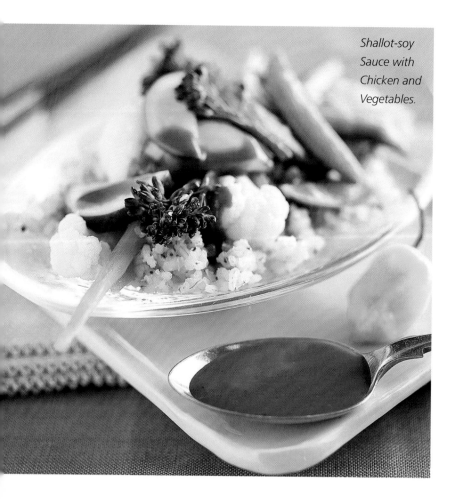

*Shallot-soy
Sauce with
Chicken and
Vegetables.*

Dinner

Shallot-Soy Sauce with Chicken and Vegetables
Heat 2 teaspoons sesame oil in a large skillet over medium-high heat. Add ½ skinless, boneless chicken breast (4 ounces) and sauté 2–3 minutes per side until golden. Add 1 minced shallot and cook 1 minute. Add ½ cup reduced-sodium chicken broth and 1 tablespoon reduced-sodium soy sauce and bring to a simmer. Simmer 5 minutes until chicken is cooked through. Top with 1 tablespoon chopped fresh cilantro before serving.

1 cup steamed green beans

¾ cup cooked wild rice

Whole-Grain Roll with Rosemary Olive Oil
Combine 2 teaspoons olive oil and ½ teaspoon minced fresh rosemary. Serve alongside one whole-grain roll (2 ounces).

8 ounces water

Dessert

Peach-Vanilla Smoothie
Combine in a blender: ½ cup fat-free vanilla frozen yogurt, ½ cup nonfat milk, 1 cup frozen peach slices, and ½ teaspoon vanilla extract. Puree until smooth.

day three

Nutrition Score: 2,220 calories, 27% fat (67 g: 14 g saturated), 54% carbohydrates (300 g), 19% protein (105 g), 36 g fiber, 1,146 mg calcium, 17 mg iron, 2,131 mg sodium

Breakfast

2 scrambled eggs (scrambled in 2 teaspoons olive oil)

1 slice whole-grain toast with 2 teaspoons fruit preserves

½ pink grapefruit

4 ounces calcium-fortified orange juice

8 ounces water

Midmorning Snack

1 cup low-fat fruit yogurt topped with 2 tablespoons pistachio nuts

1 cup red grapes

8 ounces water

Lunch

Apple-Chicken Salad

Combine in a bowl: ½ cooked, cubed skinless chicken breast (3 ounces), 1 diced Granny Smith apple, 2 tablespoons fat-free mayonnaise, ½ teaspoon curry powder, and ¼ teaspoon ground black pepper. Mix well. Spoon mixture into one whole-wheat pita pocket.

1 cup reduced-sodium tomato soup

8 ounces water

Midafternoon Snack

1 rye crispbread cracker with ¼ cup low-fat cottage cheese

2 plums

8 ounces water

Dinner

Roasted Halibut with Spicy Tomato and Green Olive Sauce

Combine in a bowl: ½ cup diced tomatoes, 2 tablespoons sliced green olives, and ½ teaspoon hot sauce. Place one 5-ounce halibut fillet in a shallow baking dish and brush the surface with 2 teaspoons olive oil. Season both sides with black pepper. Top fish with tomato mixture. Bake at 400°F for 15 minutes until fish is fork-tender.

Spinach with Garlic

Sauté 1 minced garlic clove in 2 teaspoons olive oil for 1 minute. Add 4 cups fresh spinach leaves, cover, and steam 30 seconds until spinach wilts.

½ cup cooked brown rice mixed with 2 tablespoons chopped pecans

8 ounces water

Dessert

1 cup cubed cantaloupe

day four

Nutrition Score: 2,046 calories, 20% fat (45 g: 13 g saturated), 64% carbohydrates (327 g), 16% protein (82 g), 49 g fiber, 1,236 mg calcium, 26 mg iron, 2,261 mg sodium

Breakfast

1 cup Bran Flakes cereal with ¾ cup nonfat milk

1 cup fresh or frozen cherries

8 ounces grapefruit juice

8 ounces water

Midmorning Snack

½ whole-wheat pita with 2 tablespoons prepared hummus

2 kiwis

8 ounces water

Lunch

Salami Sandwich

Top 1 slice whole-grain bread with 1 teaspoon spicy brown mustard. Top with 1 ounce light salami (Louis Rich Turkey Salami or Gallo Lite Dry Italian Salami), 2 ounces reduced-sodium provolone cheese, and 3 cucumber slices. Top with second slice of bread.

1 cup chopped Romaine lettuce with ¼ cup sliced pickled beets and 1 tablespoon fat-free French or Thousand Island dressing

1 cup cubed mango

8 ounces water

Midafternoon Snack

10 baby carrots with 1 tablespoon fat-free ranch dressing

1 pear

8 ounces water

Dinner

Grilled Shrimp with Fresh Nectarine Salsa

Preheat outdoor grill, stove-top grill pan, or broiler. In a medium bowl, combine 1 diced nectarine, 1 tablespoon chopped fresh cilantro, 2 teaspoons minced red onion, and 1 tablespoon fresh lime juice. Mix well. Season to taste with salt and black pepper. Set aside. Brush 4 ounces of peeled and deveined shrimp with 2 teaspoons olive oil and season with salt and black pepper. Grill or broil 3–5 minutes per side until fork-tender. Serve shrimp with salsa spooned over top.

½ cup cooked whole-wheat couscous mixed with 2 tablespoons toasted pine nuts (toast nuts in a hot, dry skillet over medium-high heat for 2–3 minutes until golden)

1 cup steamed snap peas tossed with 2 teaspoons sesame oil

8 ounces water

Dessert

Strawberry Shortcake

Top 1 slice fat-free pound cake (1 ounce) with 1 cup sliced strawberries. Top with second (1-ounce) slice of cake. Sift 1 teaspoon confectioners' sugar over top.

day five

Nutrition Score: 2,028 calories, 20% fat (45 g: 8 g saturated), 61% carbohydrates (309 g), 19% protein (96 g), 48 g fiber, 1,094 mg calcium, 16 mg iron, 588 mg sodium

Breakfast

Cinnamon-Nut Oats

Combine in a microwave-safe bowl: 1 cup nonfat milk, ½ cup rolled oats, 1 tablespoon chopped walnuts, and ½ teaspoon ground cinnamon. Cover with plastic wrap and microwave on high 2–3 minutes, or until liquid is absorbed.

1 cup cubed honeydew melon

8 ounces water

Midmorning Snack

1 cup cubed watermelon

¼ cup sunflower seeds

8 ounces water

Lunch

Grouper with Tomato-Basil Sauce

Place a 5-ounce grouper fillet in a microwave-safe dish. Season both sides with salt and black pepper. Top fish with 1 diced tomato and 2 tablespoons chopped fresh basil. Cover with plastic wrap and microwave on high 3 minutes until fish is fork-tender.

2 cups mixed baby lettuce with 2 tablespoons fat-free pepper-corn dressing

1 whole-grain roll (2 ounces) with 2 tablespoons apple butter

8 ounces water

Midafternoon Snack

1 pear

8 ounces calcium-fortified orange or cranberry juice

8 ounces water

Pork Medallions with Cranberry Chutney and Barley.

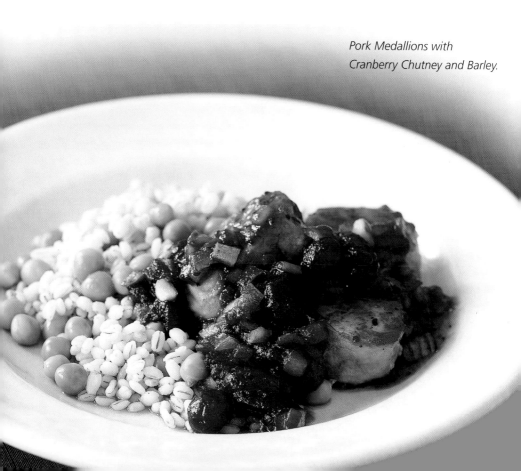

Dinner

Pork Medallions with Cranberry Chutney and Barley
In a medium saucepan over high heat, bring 1 cup water to a
boil. Add ⅓ cup quick-cooking barley, cover, reduce heat to
medium-low, and simmer 8 minutes. Add 1 cup frozen green
peas, and cook 2 more minutes until liquid is absorbed and barley is tender. Season to taste with salt and black pepper. Meanwhile, heat 2 teaspoons olive oil in a large skillet over medium-
high heat. Season both sides of 1 boneless pork loin chop
(4 ounces) with salt and black pepper and add to skillet. Sauté
2 minutes per side until golden brown. Remove pork from skillet (reserve oil in pan) and set aside. To the same pan, add ¼
cup minced onion and sauté 2 minutes. Add ⅓ cup canned cranberry sauce, 1 tablespoon cider vinegar, and ¼ teaspoon ground
ginger and bring to a simmer. Return pork to pan and simmer
2 minutes until cooked through. Serve pork and cranberry chutney with barley on the side.

8 ounces water

Dessert

1 cup each cubed pineapple and papaya

day six

Nutrition Score: 1,902 calories, 18% fat (38 g: 7 g saturated), 64% carbohydrates
(304 g), 18% protein (86 g), 36 g fiber, 916 mg calcium, 16 mg iron, 2,398 mg sodium

Breakfast

Banana-Strawberry Smoothie
Combine in a blender: 1 banana, 1 cup frozen strawberries, and
½ cup calcium-fortified orange juice. Puree until smooth.

2 slices whole-grain toast with 4 teaspoons orange marmalade

8 ounces water

Midmorning Snack

2 fennel stalks with 1 tablespoon fat-free blue cheese dressing

8 ounces water

Lunch

Toasted Pumpernickel-Salmon Salad with Dijon Vinaigrette

Place 2 cups cubed pumpernickel bread on a baking sheet and coat with olive oil spray. Bake at 400°F for 10 minutes until crisp. In a large bowl, combine one 3-ounce can water-packed salmon (drained), 2 teaspoons minced fresh dill, and 1 teaspoon drained capers. Toss. In a small bowl, whisk together 2 tablespoons red wine vinegar, 2 teaspoons olive oil, and 1 teaspoon Dijon mustard. Pour over salmon mixture and toss to coat. Add bread cubes and toss to combine. Spoon salmon mixture over 2 cups lettuce.

1 star fruit (carambola)

8 ounces water

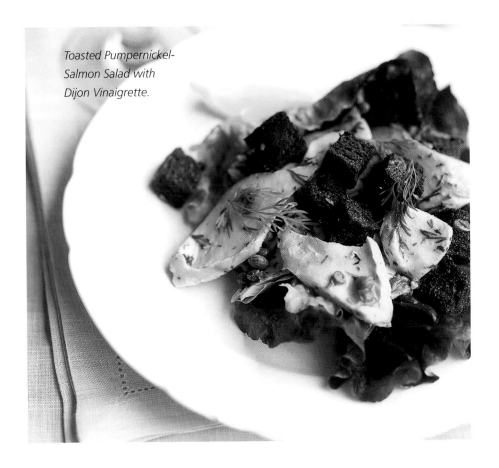

Toasted Pumpernickel-Salmon Salad with Dijon Vinaigrette.

Midafternoon Snack

Tomato-Cucumber Salad
Combine 1 sliced tomato, ½ cup sliced cucumber, 1 tablespoon balsamic vinegar, 1 teaspoon olive oil, and ¼ teaspoon dried oregano. Season to taste with salt and black pepper.

8 ounces water

Dinner

Pine-Nut Crusted Chicken Cutlets with Angel-Hair Pasta
In a shallow dish, combine 2 tablespoons seasoned dry bread crumbs and 2 teaspoons finely chopped pine nuts. Add ½ skinless, boneless chicken breast (4 ounces) and turn to coat. Heat 2 teaspoons olive oil in a large nonstick skillet over medium-high heat. Add chicken and cook 2 minutes per side until golden brown. Reduce heat to medium, cover, and cook 1–2 more minutes until chicken is cooked through. Meanwhile, toss 2 cups cooked angel hair pasta (preferably whole wheat) with 1 cup canned diced tomatoes and 1 tablespoon chopped fresh oregano or basil. Serve chicken with pasta on the side.

6 steamed asparagus spears

8 ounces water

Dessert

Mocha Malted Shake
Combine in a blender: 1 cup fat-free chocolate ice cream, 2 tablespoons prepared coffee, and 2 teaspoons malted milk powder. Puree until smooth.

day seven

Nutrition Score: 2,019 calories, 19% fat (43 g: 8 g saturated), 63% carbohydrates (318 g), 18% protein (91 g), 50 g fiber, 1,153 mg calcium, 19 mg iron, 2,010 mg sodium

Breakfast

Turkey-Cheese Breakfast Sandwich
Spray a nonstick skillet with cooking spray and place over medium-high heat. Add 1 egg and cook 2 minutes per side until yolk is cooked. Toast 1 whole-wheat English muffin. Top ½ muffin with 1 ounce fat-free American cheese and 1 ounce roasted turkey breast. Top with cooked egg and second muffin half.

4 ounces calcium-fortified orange juice

8 ounces water

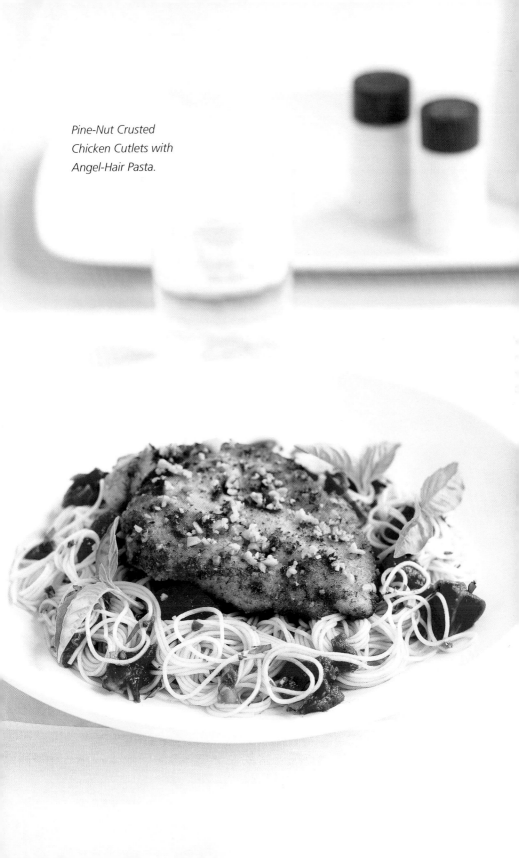

*Pine-Nut Crusted
Chicken Cutlets with
Angel-Hair Pasta.*

Midmorning Snack

⅓ cup bagel chips with 1 tablespoon prepared hummus

1 cup mixed dried fruit

8 ounces water

Lunch

Chicken Caesar Salad

In a blender or food processor, combine 1 tablespoon grated
Parmesan cheese, 2 teaspoons each Dijon mustard and olive oil,
1 teaspoon Worcestershire sauce, and 1 clove garlic. Add ⅓ cup
reduced-sodium chicken broth (or water) and puree until
smooth. Pour mixture over 2 cups chopped Romaine lettuce
and top with ½ cooked skinless, boneless chicken breast
(3 ounces) and 5 cherry tomatoes.

1 whole-grain roll (2 ounces)

8 ounces water

Midafternoon Snack

5 Greek olives (Kalamata) with 4 sesame bread sticks

1 nectarine

8 ounces water

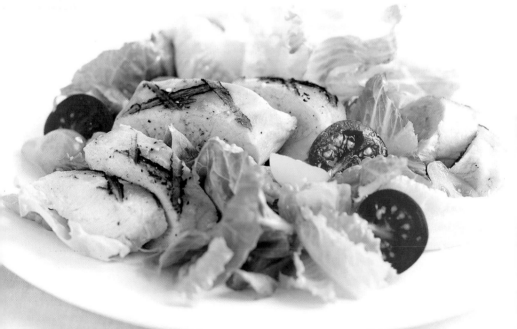

Chicken Caesar Salad.

Dinner

Spinach Linguine with Tomato-Ginger Sauce and Avocado
In a blender, combine ½ cup water, 1 tomato, ¼ cup dry sun-dried tomatoes (not oil-packed), 2 teaspoons chopped fresh ginger, 1 clove garlic, 1 tablespoon red wine vinegar, and 1 teaspoon olive oil. Process until smooth. Season to taste with salt and black pepper. Pour mixture over 1½ cups cooked spinach linguine. Top with 4 avocado slices.

1 cup steamed Brussels sprouts tossed with 2 teaspoons Dijon mustard

8 ounces water

Dessert

Broiled Apricots with Brown Sugar
Halve 2 apricots and top each half with ½ teaspoon brown sugar. Place cut side up on a baking sheet and broil 2–3 minutes until golden brown. Serve with ½ cup fat-free vanilla frozen yogurt.

week four

day one

Nutrition Score: 1,997 calories, 20% fat (44 g: 13 g saturated), 59% carbohydrates (295 g), 21% protein (105 g), 45 g fiber, 1,917 mg calcium, 21 mg iron, 2,368 mg sodium

Breakfast

1½ cups Raisin Bran cereal with 1 cup nonfat milk

1 cup blueberries

8 ounces calcium-fortified orange juice

8 ounces water

Midmorning Snack

5 reduced-fat whole-grain crackers with 2 ounces reduced-fat cheddar cheese

1 cup green grapes

8 ounces water

Lunch

Turkey BLT

Microwave 4 slices turkey bacon until crisp. Spread 2 teaspoons fat-free mayonnaise on 1 slice whole-wheat bread and top with cooked bacon, 1 lettuce leaf, and 3 tomato slices. Top with second slice of bread.

2 blood oranges or 1 regular orange

1 low-fat granola bar

8 ounces water

Midafternoon Snack

1 cup boiled soybeans (edamame)

1 peach

8 ounces herbal tea with 2 teaspoons honey

8 ounces water

Dinner

Pan-Seared Cod with Garlic-Greens, Pine Nuts, and Parmesan Polenta Toasts

Place two ½-inch-thick slices (1 ounce each) prepared polenta on a large baking sheet. Sprinkle ½ teaspoon grated Parmesan cheese on each slice. Bake at 425°F for 8–10 minutes until golden. Remove from oven and cover with foil. Meanwhile, heat 2 teaspoons olive oil in a large skillet over medium-high heat. Season both sides of one 5-ounce cod fillet with salt and black pepper and add to skillet. Cook 1–2 minutes per side until fork-tender. Remove from pan and cover with foil. To the same skillet over medium heat, add 1 minced garlic clove and 2 teaspoons pine nuts and sauté 1 minute until pine nuts are golden. Add 2 cups mustard greens, cover, and steam 30 seconds until greens are wilted. Serve garlic-greens with cod and polenta toasts.

8 ounces water

Dessert

Sautéed Banana with Brown Sugar

Combine 1 tablespoon water and 2 teaspoons light brown sugar in a large nonstick skillet. Set pan over high heat and cook until sugar melts. Add one sliced banana and cook until tender.

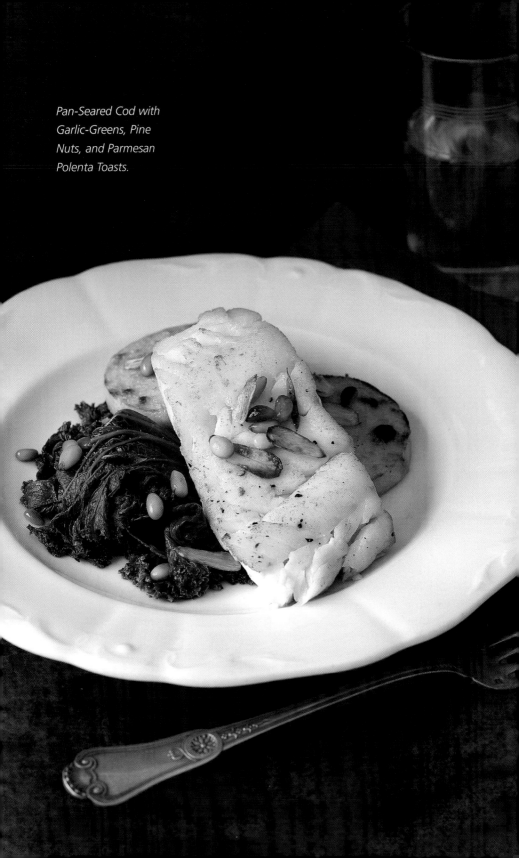

Pan-Seared Cod with
Garlic-Greens, Pine
Nuts, and Parmesan
Polenta Toasts.

10 ways to add élan to your meal plan

1. *Switch from instant to coarse oatmeal;* it's tastier and more nutritious. Soak it overnight to reduce cooking time from 30 minutes to 8. For creamier texture and a dairy serving, soak it in skim milk.

2. *Buy fruit and vegetables from farmers' markets,* or pick-your-own farms. The flavor is sweeter and fresher than most store-bought produce, plus you'll get some exercise outdoors.

3. *Cook whole grains in nonfat chicken or vegetable broth.* You'll add flavor but no fat to rice, couscous, and pasta.

4. *Experiment with gourmet vinegars;* they're as varied and complex as wines. Splashed on salads and steamed vegetables or used as a marinade, they add nonfat flavor.

5. *Create a signature dish.* Become expert at cooking one fabulous low-fat meal. You can take it to parties and potlucks and always have something healthy to eat.

6. *Grill some summer fruits,* such as chunks of pineapple and halves of slightly under-ripe apricots or peaches. Brush with apple juice, and grill until lightly browned and tender.

7. Instead of frying and sautéing, *become accomplished in healthy cooking techniques* such as steaming, stir-frying, baking, and barbecuing.

8. *Open and heat a can of low-sodium veggie-bean soup* and add three ounces of cooked, diced chicken breast or turkey sausage for a quick, well-rounded meal.

9. *Experiment with exotic tastes.* Chicken breast takes on new life when cooked in a tandoor oven at an Indian restaurant.

10. *Grow a pot of basil on a sunny windowsill.* Fresh herbs have it hands down over dried for flavor and aroma.

day two

Nutrition Score: 2,045 calories, 9% fat (20 g: 4 g saturated), 70% carbohydrates (358 g), 21% protein (107 g), 40 g fiber, 1,035 mg calcium, 13 mg iron, 2,526 mg sodium

Breakfast

2 whole-grain waffles (Eggo) with 2 tablespoons maple syrup

Creamy Chai Tea
Combine ½ cup brewed Chai tea, ½ cup nonfat milk, and
2 teaspoons honey

1 kiwi

1 star fruit (carambola)

8 ounces water

Midmorning Snack

1 cup cubed pineapple

8 ounces water

Lunch

1¼ cups black bean chili (Health Valley)

1 whole-grain roll (2 ounces)

1 cup chopped Bibb lettuce with ¼ cup shredded red cabbage
and 2 tablespoons fat-free Italian or blue cheese dressing

1 papaya topped with 2 teaspoons fresh lime juice

8 ounces water

Midafternoon Snack

½ cup low-fat cottage cheese mixed with 1/2 teaspoon salt-free
seasoning (Mrs. Dash Garlic-Herb)

2 fennel stalks

5 baby carrots

8 ounces water

Dinner

Poached Salmon with Lemon-Caper Sauce

Place one 5-ounce salmon fillet in a large saucepan. Pour over water to cover. Bring to a boil, then immediately remove from heat. Let stand 10 minutes. For sauce, whisk together ¼ cup fat-free sour cream and 2 teaspoons each fresh lemon juice and drained capers. Season to taste with salt and black pepper. Spoon sauce over drained salmon.

½ cup cooked quinoa

1 cup steamed spinach

Oven-Roasted Tomato

Halve one tomato and place cut side up on a baking sheet. Sprinkle the top with salt and black pepper. Bake at 400°F for 10 minutes until tender.

8 ounces water

Dessert

1-ounce slice angel food cake with 2 tablespoons orange marmalade

day three

Nutrition Score: 2,057 calories, 26% fat (59 g: 10 g saturated), 53% carbohydrates (273 g), 21% protein (108 g), 51 g fiber, 915 mg calcium, 24 mg iron, 2,384 mg sodium

Breakfast

Tex-Mex Scrambled Tofu

Combine in a bowl: 3 ounces diced firm tofu, 1 cup diced tomatoes (fresh or canned), 2 teaspoons chopped fresh cilantro, and ½ teaspoon each chili powder and ground cumin. Sauté mixture in a hot skillet for 5 minutes, stirring frequently until mixture thickens.

1 slice whole-wheat toast with 2 teaspoons fruit preserves

8 ounces water

Midmorning Snack

¼ cup dry roasted peanuts with ¼ cup raisins

1 cup blackberries or raspberries

8 ounces water

Lunch

Cobb Salad

Top 2 cups chopped Romaine lettuce with 2 ounces sliced turkey breast, ½ cup sliced cucumber, 5 baby carrots, ¼ cup cubed avocado, 1 tablespoon crumbled blue cheese, and 3 jumbo black olives. Top with 2 tablespoons fat-free dressing (any flavor).

Mexican Rice and Beans

Combine in a microwave-safe bowl: 1 cup water, ¾ cup instant brown rice, ⅓ cup canned black beans (rinsed), and ½ teaspoon ground cumin. Cover with plastic wrap and microwave on high 3–5 minutes until liquid is absorbed.

1 cup strawberries

8 ounces water

Midafternoon Snack

1 low-fat granola bar

4 ounces calcium-fortified orange or cranberry juice

8 ounces water

Dinner

Chicken Pot Stickers

In a large bowl, combine 4 ounces ground chicken breast, 1 chopped green onion, 1 tablespoon reduced-sodium soy sauce, and salt and black pepper to taste. Mix well and divide mixture into 2 equal portions. Place each portion on the center of one egg roll wrapper. Moisten edges of wrappers with water and pull up corners so they meet in the center. Pinch together edges to seal. Heat 2 teaspoons sesame oil in a large nonstick skillet over medium heat. Add stuffed wrappers and sauté 2 minutes until golden brown on the bottom. Add ½ cup reduced-sodium chicken broth, cover, and steam 5 minutes until chicken is cooked through.

2 cups steamed broccoli

½ cup shredded green cabbage with 2 tablespoons fat-free ranch dressing

8 ounces water

Dessert

½ cup fat-free mint chocolate chip ice cream or frozen yogurt

1 cup strawberries

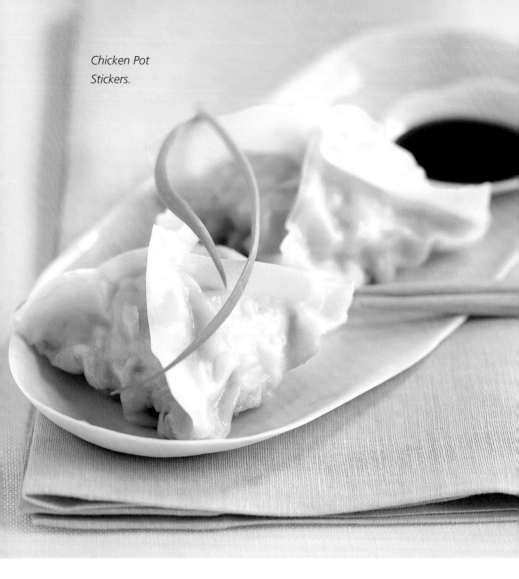

Chicken Pot Stickers.

day four

Nutrition Score: 2,083 calories, 13% fat (30 g: 7 g saturated), 70% carbohydrates (365 g), 17% protein (89 g), 48 g fiber, 1,146 mg calcium, 16 mg iron, 1,629 mg sodium

Breakfast

¾ cup low-fat granola with ¾ cup nonfat milk

2 cups cubed cantaloupe

8 ounces water

Midmorning Snack

2 plums

8 ounces water

Lunch

1 cup vegetarian chili

1 whole-grain roll (2 ounces)

2 cups chopped Bibb lettuce with ¼ cup sliced pickled beets and 2 tablespoons fat-free Italian or blue cheese dressing

1 papaya topped with 2 teaspoons fresh lime juice

8 ounces water

Midafternoon Snack

6-ounce container soy yogurt topped with 1 tablespoon honey crunch wheat germ

8 ounces water

Dinner

Grilled Tuna with Fresh Peach Salsa
Preheat outdoor grill, stove-top grill pan, or broiler. In a medium bowl, combine 1 diced peach, 1 tablespoon chopped fresh cilantro, and 2 teaspoons each minced red onion and fresh lime juice. Season to taste with salt and black pepper. Set aside. Brush one 5-ounce tuna steak with 2 teaspoons olive oil and season with salt and black pepper. Grill or broil 3–5 minutes per side until fork-tender. Serve tuna with salsa spooned over top.

½ cup cooked whole-wheat couscous mixed with 2 teaspoons pistachio nuts

6 steamed asparagus spears

8 ounces water

Dessert

Blueberry Parfait
Layer in a tall glass: 1 cup low-fat vanilla yogurt and 1 cup blueberries.

day five

Nutrition Score: 2,053 calories, 21% fat (48 g: 10 g saturated), 63% carbohydrates (323 g), 16% protein (82 g), 30 g fiber, 844 mg calcium, 16 mg iron, 2,171 mg sodium

Breakfast

3 scrambled egg whites (scrambled in 1 teaspoon olive oil)

1 toasted oat bran English muffin with 2 teaspoons fruit preserves

1 cup cubed watermelon

4 ounces low-sodium vegetable juice

8 ounces water

Midmorning Snack

Trail Mix
Combine ¼ cup each Honey Bunches of Oats cereal and minced dried fruit bits and 2 teaspoons slivered almonds.

8 ounces water

Lunch

Orange-Glazed Chicken
Coat ½ skinless, boneless chicken breast (4 ounces) with a mixture of 2 tablespoons orange marmalade and 1 teaspoon reduced-sodium soy sauce. Transfer chicken to a baking sheet. Bake at 400°F for 25 minutes until cooked through.

8 endive leaves topped with 1 tablespoon crumbled blue cheese and 1 tablespoon fat-free Italian dressing

2 reduced-fat whole-grain crackers

4 ounces calcium-fortified grapefruit juice

8 ounces water

Midafternoon Snack

2 cups grapes

¼ cup roasted pumpkin seeds

8 ounces water

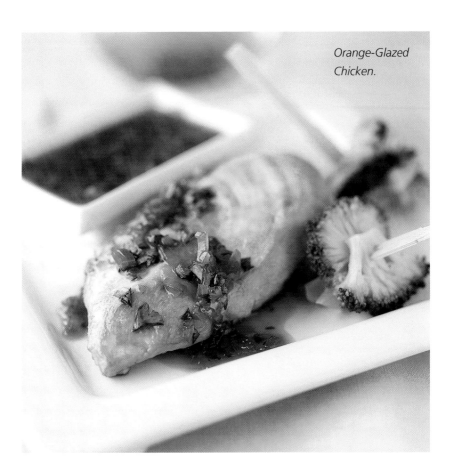

Orange-Glazed Chicken.

Dinner

Spicy Peanut Sauce with Vegetables and Brown Rice

In a small saucepan, whisk together ½ cup reduced-sodium chicken broth, 1 tablespoon each reduced-fat peanut butter and hoisin sauce, and 1 teaspoon hot sauce. Set pan over medium-low heat and simmer 10 minutes, stirring frequently with a wire whisk. Meanwhile, combine ¾ cup instant brown rice and ¾ cup water in a microwave-safe dish. Cover with plastic wrap and cook on high 3–5 minutes until liquid is absorbed. Toss rice with 2 cups mixed vegetables (such as broccoli florets, sliced zucchini, baby carrots, snap peas, and cauliflower florets) and spoon peanut sauce over top.

8 ounces water

Dessert

1-ounce slice fat-free chocolate loaf cake (Entenmanns) with 1 cup raspberries and 2 teaspoons chocolate syrup

8 ounces nonfat milk

day six

Nutrition Score: 2,096 calories, 16% fat (37 g: 7 g saturated), 67% carbohydrates (351 g), 17% protein (89 g), 47 g fiber, 1,038 mg calcium, 16 mg iron, 2,482 mg sodium

Breakfast

Cantaloupe-Strawberry Smoothie
Combine in a blender: 1 cup each cubed cantaloupe, strawberries, and low-fat strawberry yogurt; and 1 teaspoon wheat germ. Puree until smooth.

½ whole-wheat pita with 2 teaspoons prepared hummus

8 ounces herbal tea

8 ounces water

Midmorning Snack

½ cup golden raisins with ¼ cup pecans

8 ounces water

Lunch

Soy BLT
Microwave 3 slices soy bacon (Lightlife Smart) until crisp. Spread 2 teaspoons fat-free mayonnaise on one slice of whole-wheat bread. Top with cooked bacon, 1 lettuce leaf, and 3 tomato slices. Top with second slice of bread.

1 sliced mango

8 ounces water

Midafternoon Snack

5 reduced-fat whole-grain crackers with 1 ounce smoked part-skim mozzarella cheese

8 ounces water

Dinner

Sundried Tomato Sauce with Bay Scallops

Combine in a blender: ½ cup sundried tomatoes (not oil-packed), 1 cup reduced-sodium chicken broth, 1 clove garlic, and 2 teaspoons balsamic vinegar. Puree until smooth. Transfer mixture to a medium saucepan and set pan over medium heat. Simmer 5 minutes. Add ¼ pound bay scallops, cover, and simmer 5 minutes until scallops are tender. Remove from heat and stir in 1 tablespoon chopped fresh basil. Season to taste with salt and black pepper. Serve over 2 cups cooked whole-wheat pasta spirals.

2 cups steamed broccoli tossed with 2 tablespoons cooked soybeans and 1 teaspoon olive oil. Season to taste with salt and black pepper.

8 ounces water

Dessert

1 frozen banana with 2 tablespoons warmed chocolate syrup

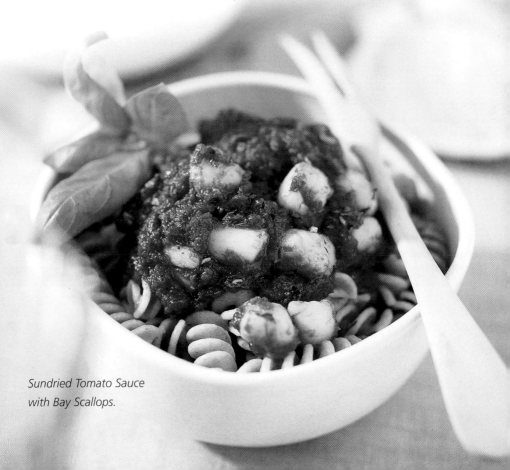

Sundried Tomato Sauce with Bay Scallops.

day seven

Nutrition Score: 2,070 calories, 12% fat (28 g: 6 g saturated), 72% carbohydrates (373 g), 16% protein (83 g), 58 g fiber, 1,158 mg calcium, 24 mg iron, 1,504 mg sodium

Breakfast

1 cup cooked hot wheat cereal with 2 minced dried plums

½ grapefruit

8 ounces nonfat milk or calcium-fortified vanilla soy milk

8 ounces water

Midmorning Snack

2 slices whole-grain bread with 2 tablespoons apple butter

2 clementines or 1 orange

8 ounces water

Lunch

Chicken Wrap
Top one 8-inch spinach or whole-wheat tortilla with 2 tea-spoons honey mustard. Top with 2 ounces roasted chicken breast, 1 ounce reduced-fat Monterey Jack cheese, ½ cup water-cress, and 4 tomato slices. Roll up.

1 orange

8 ounces water

Midafternoon Snack

1 baked sweet potato with 1 tablespoon barbecue sauce

1 star fruit (carambola)

8 ounces water

Dinner

Kasha-Pasta Salad with Roasted Peppers and Pine Nuts
Place 1 tablespoon pine nuts in a small skillet and set pan over medium-high heat. Cook 2–3 minutes until nuts are golden brown. Set aside. In a small bowl, combine ¼ cup kasha (roasted buckwheat) and 1 egg white and stir to coat. Heat 2 teaspoons olive oil in a small saucepan over medium heat. Add kasha and cook 2–3 minutes until egg is cooked and kasha kernels sepa-rate. Add ½ cup reduced-sodium chicken broth, reduce heat to

soul food

In our zeal to eat a healthy diet, we must guard against forgetting that food is essential to life and—most of all—a pleasure. Certain foods are "soul foods," with an emotional content that goes far beyond their physical reality: the cheesecake you used to share with your high-school best friend, the spaghetti marinara from Maria's Kitchen that you fell in love over, the rice pudding your mother made when you were sick. These foods soothe us, take us back in time, and unite our bodies with our hearts and our minds.

So what can you do to recapture the inherent soul-fulfilling capacity of food? One answer can be found in the Eastern religious tradition of mindful eating. In its most literal incarnation, mindful eating involves picturing the food's transformation from golden fields of wheat to brown loaves of bread, from a black-and-white Guernsey to a pristine glass of milk or a lusty Camembert—and reflecting on the gratitude this transformation demands from us. In more down-to-earth terms, it simply means eating slowly and consciously, noticing and savoring flavors and textures, enjoying the act of eating in a way that's as far from "fast food" as it's humanly possible to get.

The Western version of soulful eating is perhaps best embodied in the old-world tradition of the Sunday dinner: wine, family, cooking, and eating together in a celebration of the pleasures of life. This food is inseparable from emotion. This is the food we cannot live without—and fats, protein, and carbohydrates have nothing to do with it.

low, cover, and simmer 7 minutes until liquid is absorbed.
Toss with 1 cup cooked whole-wheat pasta spirals, 1 cup diced roasted red peppers (from water-packed jar), and 1 tablespoon each balsamic vinegar and chopped fresh parsley. Toss to combine, and season to taste with salt and black pepper. Top with pine nuts before serving.

8 ounces water

Dessert

1 cup chocolate sorbet with 1 biscotti cookie
1 cup blackberries or blueberries

Mistake to Avoid:
Although soy in the form of soybeans, tofu, and soy milk is healthy, soybean oil—especially hydrogenated or partially hydrogenated oil—is not! In most Americans' diets, hydrogenated oils are the primary source of trans fatty acids, which damage the cardiovascular system. Trans fats in the form of hydrogenated oils are common in fast foods such as french fries and prepackaged foods (snack cakes and the like).

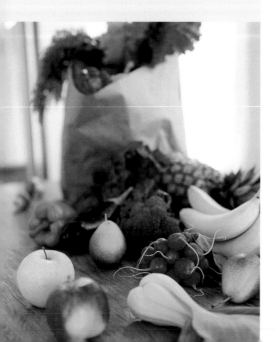

shop right, shave calories

Once you've followed our eating plan for four weeks, you'll get to know which foodstuffs and serving sizes make up a healthy diet, and you'll be able to create your own menus. Stocking up on fresh, low-fat, high-fiber foods is key to keeping you on track. When nutrient-rich food is easily accessible, you're likely to actually use what's on hand. In other words, if you don't keep those Fatty-Cheesy-Salty Snacks in your cupboard, you'll probably reach for the whole-grain crackers and reduced-fat peanut butter instead.

So, healthy eating starts in the grocery store. You need to load your cabinets, refrigerator, and freezer with the best choices the market has to offer. As a bonus, you'll find that your tab is lower at the checkout stand. Shopping for a simple, plant-based diet is often less expensive than traditional American staples such as red meat, butter, cheese, high-sugar cereals, and processed snacks.

Still, you need to be an aware consumer if you're going to steer clear of those staples presented so enticingly in the store. At one time, nutritionists recommended shopping the perimeter of the market

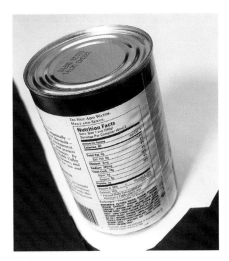

If you know how to decipher them, food labels can help you control fat and calorie intake while getting the nutrients you need.

where you would find the produce section, the dairy case, and the bakery. The center aisles, chock full of processed foods, were places best avoided. But savvy retailers are on to us. Now you'll find, for instance, dessert toppings and high-fat salad dressings nestled right next to fruit and veggies in the produce section. Keeping a detailed shopping list will help you cut down on impulse buying when you run across these strategically placed tempting items.

You also should become an avid label reader. Products with names that include words such as *light, natural,* and *healthy* often don't have any of those attributes. Scanning the nutrition label and the ingredients list will confirm that fact.

Nutrition labels can be your friend when it comes to maintaining a healthy diet, but studies have shown that many people don't know how (or don't bother) to decipher them. They're broken down into three sections:

1. *Top* (serving size and number of servings): The biggest mistake you can make is assuming that there's one serving in the package. If you don't notice that one serving is one cup, and there are two cups in the box or can, you'll double the calories and fat you get. Labels will often say "about" two servings in the package, so it's up to you to measure out the serving size.

2. *Middle* (amount per serving and percentage of daily values): Here you get to see those important fat, cholesterol, sodium, fiber, and sugar amounts. Note how much each element contributes to the recommended daily maximum. Label figures are always based on a 2,000-calorie-per-day diet.

If you're on a different calorie count, there's a way to formulate the percentages. But most of us aren't going to do the math. Just be aware that if two grams of fat equals 3 percent of the recommended daily value of fat for a 2,000-calorie diet, it will contribute a slightly bigger percentage to an 1,800-calorie diet.

3. *Bottom* (vitamins A and C, calcium, iron): Compare the percentages of each serving to your total recommended daily intake (for a printable list of recommended daily amounts, go to **www.nal.usda.gov/fnic/dga/rda.pdf**). While it's not practical to do this for every food you eat, it's a good way to keep track if, say, you're trying to increase your calcium intake.

The ingredients list is just as important. This is where you can determine if the product is loaded with trans fats. At some point, the government might include trans fats on the nutritional label as it now does with saturated fats, but in the meantime, you need to look for—and avoid—them in the form of hydrogenated or partially hydrogenated oils.

One of the great innovations in recent years is that most major food corporations now have Web-sites where you can check the nutritional breakdowns of their products. This means you can do your comparison shopping of breakfast cereals or soups before you ever leave home.

Quick Tip: *Studies show that people who drink five or more eight-ounce cups of water a day have a lower risk of developing breast cancer and other serious healthy problems. But you don't have to limit yourself to plain water. You can include soups, juices, and herbal teas in your fluid intake. Alcoholic and caffeinated beverages (including sodas such as Pepsi, Coca-Cola, Dr. Pepper, and Mountain Dew) count half or less, though, because alcohol and caffeine have a diuretic effect.*

an insider's guide
to the grocery store

Here are some tips for successfully navigating the grocery store:

bread, cereals, and grains

- Just because bread is brown doesn't make it whole grain. Wheat flour—even enriched or fortified wheat flour—is not whole grain. The first ingredient should *say* whole grain, whole wheat, or rye. Opt for breads with two or more grams of fiber and 70 to 90 calories per slice.

- Choose breakfast cereals that are high in fiber and low in sugar. A serving of Kellogg's All-Bran has 80 calories, 10 grams of fiber, and 6 grams of sugar; a serving of Kellogg's Cocoa Krispies has 120 calories, 1 gram of fiber, and 14 grams of sugar. The comparison is not quite equitable, as a serving of All-Bran is ½ cup, while a serving of Cocoa Krispies is ¾ cup. See what we mean about reading labels? Still, even after you do the math, the All-Bran comes out ahead nutritionally.

- Crackers are all too easy to nibble on and can be deceptively high in fat, so buy brands such as reduced-fat Triscuits or nonfat Ry Krisps.

- If you're turned off by brown rice because it takes longer to cook than white, keep a couple of boxes of quick-cooking brown rice on hand.

- Experiment with grains such as buckwheat groats (kasha), quinoa (pronounced *keen-wa*), bulgur, and barley.

- When you put tortillas on your shopping list, make them whole wheat or corn. Read the label to make sure they're not laden with lard.

- Keep whole-wheat spaghetti or pasta spirals on hand. Pasta varieties such as spinach or sun-dried tomato have some added flavor, but nothing in the way of added nutrition.

beans and legumes

- Put off by beans because of all that overnight soaking? No problem. Stock up on canned pinto beans, garbanzo beans (chickpeas), cannellini beans, black beans, kidney beans, lentils, and black-eyed peas.

- Peanuts are also legumes, but nutritionally, they're more like nuts (high in fat). Look for reduced-fat peanut butter.

dairy, soy, and eggs

- Cheese is a great source of calcium (except cottage cheese), but hard cheeses are packed with fat grams (three ounces of cheddar can have 28 grams of fat, 18 grams saturated). Look for reduced-fat brands. Opt for soft cheeses such as ricotta and farmer, which are made from skim or part-skim milk. Strongly flavored cheeses such as Parmesan and Romano are a good bet, as a little grating adds a lot of taste.

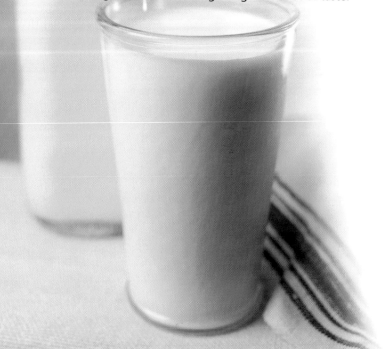

- Stick to skim or low-fat (1-percent) milk. The Food and Drug Administration (FDA) defines "low-fat" as containing three or fewer grams of fat per serving. That lets out 2-percent milk, which contains 5 grams per serving.

- Buy eight-ounce containers of low-fat, plain yogurt. Sugar content of flavored yogurts can be as high as a candy bar. Low-fat vanilla ice cream or frozen yogurt make good desserts.

- Fortified soy products—milk, yogurt, and cheese—are good substitutes for dairy, and nutritious in their own right. If you haven't liked them in the past, give soy products another chance from time to time—manufacturers are constantly improving the taste and texture of soy foods. You can also get your soy ration from frozen soybeans (edamame).

- To be sure of getting fresh eggs, buy six at a time. If you're watching fat consumption, get a six-ounce container of refrigerated egg whites, or use egg substitutes.

Quick Tip: *Don't be afraid of eggs! Healthy women can eat up to seven eggs a week without worry. In addition to high-quality protein, eggs contain five grams of healthy fat and only two grams of saturated fat. Plus, they're a good source of minerals and vitamins, including zinc and vitamins A, D, and E.*

nuts/seeds/oils

- Stick to raw, unsalted nuts. Your staples should include almonds, walnuts, and tahini (sesame paste). If you buy nuts in bulk, keep them in the refrigerator for freshness: The oils in nuts can go rancid.

- Olive oil is a must, but so is canola oil. Buy eight-ounce bottles to maintain freshness.

produce

- Remember, you're buying enough to provide eight servings of fruit and vegetables a day, so fresh produce will take up most of the room in your shopping cart. Go for a seasonal mix of produce, being sure to buy a variety of colors, especially dark ones, to maximize your intake of vitamins and phytochemicals.

- *Best-bet vegetables:* cabbage, broccoli, sweet potatoes, Swiss chard, kale, carrots, onions, winter squashes, garlic, bell peppers, fennel, red leaf lettuce, tomatoes, spinach, and collard greens.

- *Best-bet fruits:* apples, oranges, pink grapefruit, blueberries, strawberries, raspberries, mangos, papayas, red grapes, kiwis, cantaloupe, honeydew melon, dried fruit in moderation (especially antioxidant-rich plums), and avocado (yes, they're a fruit!).

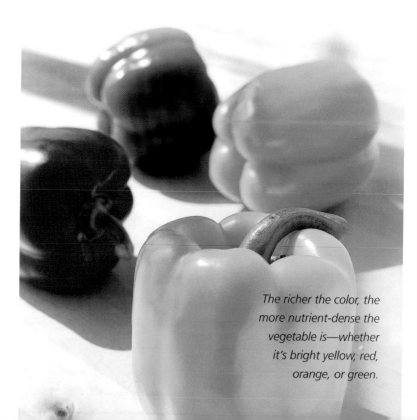

The richer the color, the more nutrient-dense the vegetable is—whether it's bright yellow, red, orange, or green.

frozen foods

- Frozen produce is often as nutritious as its fresh counterparts since it's frozen immediately after harvest.

- Frozen vegetable blends (without high-fat sauces) make planning healthy meals a breeze. Keep a 16-ounce bag of mixed vegetables for quick stir-fry dishes.

- Frozen fruits can go into smoothies, muffins, and quick breads. Toss some 16-ounce bags of frozen peaches, berries, or cherries into your cart.

- Bags of frozen, skinless chicken breasts can form the basis for a speedy, nutritious dish. Defrost in the microwave, then stir-fry, grill, or simmer in soups—they're a quick fix.

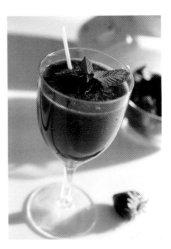

Frozen fruit is great for desserts that are short on prep time and long on taste and nutrition.

- When time's really at a premium, healthy frozen breakfasts such as Eggo Nutri-grain Whole Wheat Waffles, and savory entrees (served with extra vegetables and fruit) such as Weight Watchers Smart Ones, Healthy Choice, and Lean Cuisine can save the day.

fish

- Fresh, frozen, or canned, seafood has all the nutritional benefits of meat and poultry without the saturated fat.

- Make your choice from fatty fish, such as salmon, albacore tuna, sardines, and herrings that are all rich in omega-3 fatty acids. Avoid fish canned in oil. Instead, buy it in water or tomato sauce.

- Other types of fish and shellfish are good sources of low-fat protein, and are less likely to be tainted with mercury and pesticide residues.

meat and poultry

- White-meat poultry—essentially, the breast—is lower in fat than dark. Don't be fooled by buying packages of ground turkey meat thinking that it's healthier than ground beef. Read the nutrition label carefully, as often it contains dark meat and fat, and is as fatty or more so than reduced-fat ground beef.

- For your occasional meat treat, look for lean cuts of beef round loin, sirloin, chuck arm, pork tenderloin, and center loin. Trim visible fat before cooking.

staples

You're going to need these taste boosters to keep on hand: salt and pepper; fat-free salad dressing; ground spices such as cumin, coriander, chili, cinnamon, allspice, and nutmeg; curry powder; tomato paste; vinegars such as cider, red wine, rice, and balsamic; mustards; low-fat chicken and vegetable broth; capers; Kalamata olives; a jar of roasted red peppers; sesame seeds; maple syrup; and unsweetened cocoa powder.

Mistake to Avoid:

Polyunsaturated oils such as corn, soybean, and safflower are good for you, right? Wrong! Omega-3 fatty acids found in fish, walnuts, and canola oil are health-promoting. Both the American Heart Association and the American Cancer Society urge you to limit other polyunsaturated fats to no more than 10 percent of your total daily calories.

the program in action

Food controlled almost every aspect of the first 20 years of Debra Orringer's life. "I often ate because I was bored or upset, not because I was truly in need of nourishment," she says. Since she wasn't very active, the weight piled on, and by the time she turned 15, she weighed 250 pounds.

Debra, a Florida native, got a wake-up call to become healthy the summer before her junior year in college. She spent the break working for the university painting and preparing dorm rooms for incoming students. "It was physically demanding work, and wearing heavy sweat pants and a baggy T-shirt in the 100-plus-degree heat left me miserable," she says. "I caught a glimpse of myself in a mirror and was disgusted with what I saw." Then and there she determined to stop complaining and lose weight.

A weight-loss counselor helped Debra get to the root of her overeating. She learned to turn to other things besides food when she was bored or upset. "I stopped thinking about food all the time and instead called a friend or took a walk," she says. She began eating smaller portions of healthful, satisfying meals, filled with whole grains, fruits, vegetables, and fat.

The counselor cautioned her against cutting fat completely out of her diet. "She said if I did, I would crave high-fat foods like cake and cookies even more, causing me to binge."

These changes, along with regular exercise, which Debra did in the form of step aerobics and weight training, kick-started her weight loss. She worked out in the morning, which inspired her to eat wholesome food throughout the day. "I lost 50 pounds during the first year, and my self-esteem soared."

She continued to lose weight for the next several years and lost 40 more pounds. "Eating to fuel my body, rather than soothe my emotions, became second nature," says Debra, now 30. She has also become an athlete and has participated in several triathlons.

"I bought a bikini for the first time in my life last summer and loved how I felt when I wore it out in public. Healthful eating and regular exercise now have become lifelong habits, and I can't imagine living any other way."

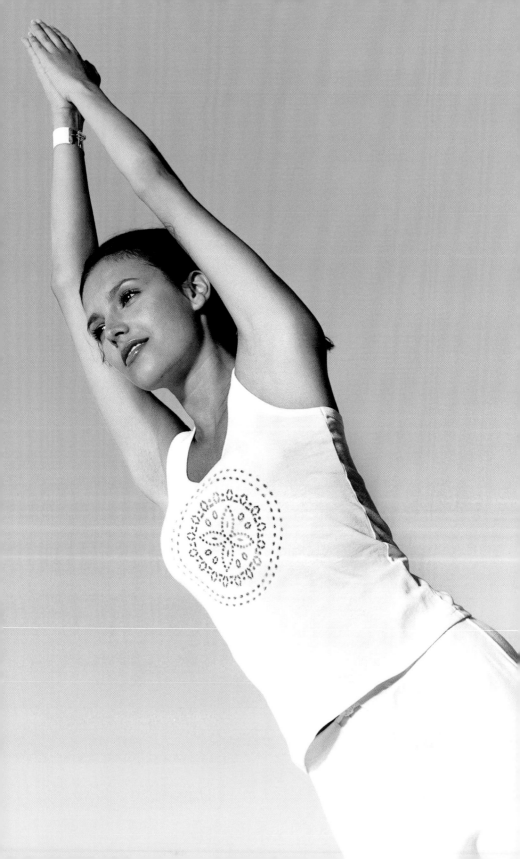

chapter three
your spirituality

Quick Tip: *Revel in silence. Don't always automatically turn on the TV when you get home, or the radio as soon as you get in car. Without distractions, you can tune in to the soothing sounds of nature.*

what you'll learn

Shape's approach to spirituality is to help you go beyond simple mental and physical fitness to being truly healthy, which requires nurturing and developing your spiritual self as well.

Using this chapter, you'll improve your spiritual fitness and health by using one or all of *Shape*'s four-week plans to:

- find new ways to connect with others and strengthen social ties
- explore volunteer opportunities to find one that's just right for you
- renew your relationship with nature by getting outdoors more
- discover what kind of meditation practice works for you
- keep a journal to learn more about yourself and what you believe
- enjoy a fresh approach to exercise that's mindful, based on tuning in to your body and its sensations

how you'll do it

A fit body is only one part of the equation for shaping a healthy life. The path to it is an internal journey as well as an external one. Nurturing your spirituality can profoundly affect your health and provide the serenity and self-awareness that the pace of our technology-driven society, information overload, and materialistic values often erode.

"Over the past few decades, we've enjoyed a steady level of prosperity in this country and have focused on all the material goods that go along with success," says Shana Aborn, a magazine editor in New York City, who rediscovered her roots in Judaism and subsequently authored *30 Days to a More Spiritual Life*. "But people are beginning to realize that this is not what life is all about. They're starting to wonder if there's more out there for them." In the face of uncertainty and danger, too, a spiritual grounding can keep fear from overwhelming you.

All indications suggest that our spirits are hungry, and it's a perfectly human response to seek nourishment. The quest for spiritual enlighten-ment certainly has to be the oldest "new" trend ever to rock popular cul-ture. Spirituality is a hot topic on talk shows and prime-time TV. Guides to the care of the soul now fill self-help displays that once offered diet and exercise manuals. Just as the fitness craze prompted us to pay attention to our bodies, we seem to be in the midst of a spiritual awakening. The urge to feed our spirits has important health consequences, too. Spiritual health affects physical health and is an important aspect of your ability to care for yourself. By learning to love yourself, appreciate your life, feel grateful, and trust yourself, you'll become a better person, friend, partner, parent, and member of the community, as well as enjoying unique health payoffs.

But what exactly do we mean by "spirituality"? According to Timothy Freke, author of *Encyclopedia of Spirituality*, spirituality is ". . . about set-ting out on a personal search for answers to the most profound questions of life. It's a journey of awakening to who we really are." Spirituality is about finding meaning, purpose, and fulfillment in life. And this may or may not include religion. Although many people find sustenance in the val-ues, rituals, and community of their organized religion, others form a system of belief through nonreligious sources such as nature, meditation, or volunteering.

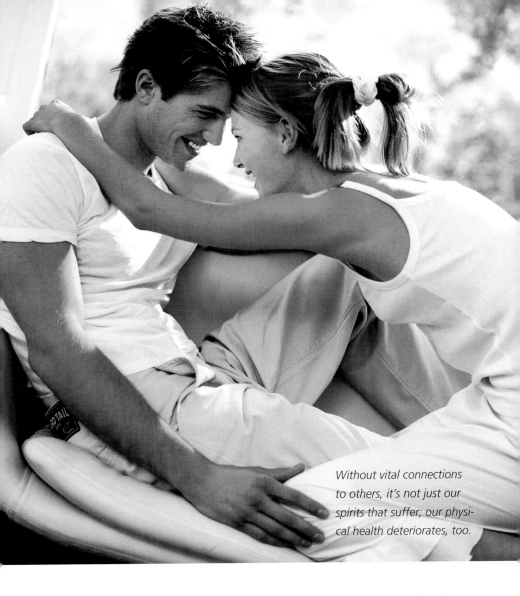

Without vital connections to others, it's not just our spirits that suffer; our physical health deteriorates, too.

Whether they do it in a cathedral or on a mountaintop, people who take time to nurture their spirituality universally describe themselves as possessing a sense of peace and wholeness, of feeling connected. Studies have found that those with a strong sense of spirituality even have better mental and physical health.

If these are the characteristics of a healthy, well-nourished spirit, the opposite is true for one that is starved. Signs that your spirit needs care may include undefined inner yearnings, a lack of joy, and feelings of being closed down and disconnected. When you don't offer nourishment to your spirit, you can suffer from a variety of physical and emotional symptoms, such as anxiety, fatigue, illness, and depression. Yet we can easily misinterpret these symptoms. We misread our spiritual hunger and feed it the wrong things: junk food, alcohol, drugs, or unhealthy relationships.

Ask yourself: Do you love your life? Are you happy to be alive? Robert Ivker, D.O., past president of the American Holistic Medical Association, states that how you respond to these questions can be a more precise barometer of your total health picture than measurements such as blood pressure and what you weigh. That's because the quality of your daily experiences and your spiritual and mental vitality affect your physiology, and so, truly influence your health.

Mistake to Avoid: *Don't beat yourself up over negative feelings such as jealousy, envy, or anger. Instead, examine those emotions neutrally and learn from them: Ask yourself what's really generating them and how you can resolve them without hurting yourself or others. Writing about them in your journal can be a powerful way to defuse the emotions and help you come up with positive actions to resolve whatever is troubling you.*

body and soul

In the past, the medical community has disregarded and misinterpreted the spiritual aspects of our total health. But now the American Association of Medical Colleges (AAMC) in Washington, D.C., has added "social and spiritual competency" to its curriculum guidelines, identifying it as a skill that all medical-school graduates should possess. Over 70 American medical schools now teach new doctors to respect patients' social and spiritual lives.

are you starving your soul?

Are you leaving time in your life for nourishing spirituality and emotional intimacy with your buddies, your spouse, and your children? Take this quiz to determine where you stand.

YES NO

___ ✓ 1. I make time for prayer, meditation, or reflection on a regular basis.

✓ ___ 2. I listen to and act on my intuition.

✓ ___ 3. I'm grateful for the blessings in my life.

___ ✓ 4. I observe a day of rest away from work, dedicated to nurturing myself and my family.

✓ ___ 5. I have the ability to forgive myself and others.

✓ ___ 6. I experience intimacy, besides sex, in my committed relationships.

✓ ___ 7. I find peace and satisfaction in ordinary activities.

✓ ___ 8. I know what I believe in and could explain it to others.

✓ ___ 9. I've offered a helping hand to others in the last week.

✓ ___ 10. I've taken time to appreciate nature in the last week.

SCORING

It's impossible to calculate an RDA for spiritual nourishment. So clearly it's not feasible to say how many yes answers constitutes a spiritually fulfilling life for you. Yet we all seem to experience a greater sense of well-being when we properly feed our spirits—and an odd, empty feeling when we don't. So look at those questions to which you responded negatively, and use our four-week plans to turn each no into a yes.

spirituality and longevity

A 25-year research project has discovered that the population of the Japanese island-state of Okinawa has a higher percentage of healthy centenarians than anywhere else on Earth. True, the Okinawans eat a healthful plant-based diet and routinely incorporate physical activity into their daily lives. But spirituality also permeates all facets of Okinawans' existence. It's rooted in Taoism and its profound reverence for nature, Confucianism and its deep respect for others, and native spirituality, where elders are revered and women are the keepers of—that is, "the pray-ers" for—the spiritual bonds between modern society and all things past. Successful aging is actually celebrated with healing rituals: In one custom, ayakaru, it's said that by touching an elder, you can share in that person's good fortune, health, and long life.

The Okinawan spiritual philosophy affirms a faith in humanity, and it emphasizes both personal and group responsibilities. Okinawans believe that if someone fails, whether through bad luck or any other reason, there's an obligation on the part of others to help. There is significant research to show that these deep convictions can protect us from stress, and stress-related illness. These are concepts that we can integrate into our daily lives to maintain our physical, emotional, and spiritual health.

Some authorities still assert that matters of the soul should take precedence over concerns of the body, or vice versa. Other experts in science and medicine, however, are recognizing an amazing partnership between the physical and spiritual. According to neuroscientist Andrew Newberg, M.D., co-author of *Why God Won't Go Away: Brain Science and the Biology of Belief,* an active region in the back of the brain that processes information about space and time becomes quiet during med-

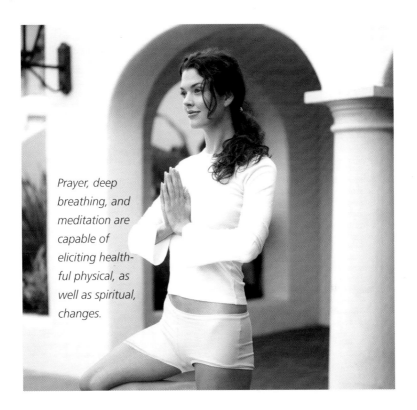

Prayer, deep breathing, and meditation are capable of eliciting healthful physical, as well as spiritual, changes.

itation. During this practice, the distinction between oneself and the surrounding universe is obliterated. Newberg and fellow researchers have come to believe that human beings are biologically wired for spirituality.

Herbert Benson, M.D., founder of the Mind/Body Institute in Boston, turned the medical community on its ear 30 years ago when he first suggested that tools of mental relaxation such as prayer and meditation could elicit a set of healthful physiological changes.

Benson has studied at length the benefits of what he calls "the Faith Factor." According to him, you can experience a deeper, more beneficial sense of relaxation if you evoke your personal beliefs. It doesn't matter whether those beliefs are secular or religious, as long as you have a guiding principle to call upon in time of need. He cites studies in which patients, drawing on their own set of beliefs as a healing tool, were able to reduce drug and alcohol dependencies, depression, anxiety, and blood pressure.

The evidence is mounting that nurturing our spirits has beneficial consequences in all aspects of our lives. And we're not limited in ways to accomplish this aim. One fascinating aspect of spirituality is that there are as many ways to explore it as there are seekers. Yet most believers— whether they observe organized religions or pursue their own interpretations of spirituality—tend to share some similar core convictions and practices. These are: the sense that each individual is part of a greater whole; the desire to help and serve others; a deep respect for nature; silence, contemplation, and reflection; examination of one's behavior and beliefs; and spiritually oriented exercise. You may already engage in some of these practices. If not, follow our four-week plan at the end of each section for enriching your spiritual health.

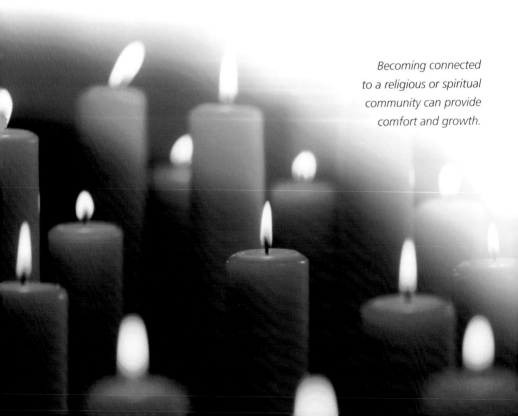

Becoming connected to a religious or spiritual community can provide comfort and growth.

connectedness

Everyone has different social needs, but it's no surprise that more and more of us find ourselves lacking the connections with others that are so vital to our spiritual health. We don't know our neighbors, we shop on the Internet and socialize via e-mail, we never seem to have enough time for our friends, we work out solo wearing headphones that keep the world out, and we jump from job to job and city to city.

We even tend to live by ourselves: The number of Americans living singly has been rising steadily since the 1980s. Our culture stresses the importance of individualism, independence, and self-reliance, but at what price? These are the very same traits that can lead to fewer contacts with other people, resulting in alienation. Without friends and loved ones to rely on, confide in, and feel totally comfortable with, it's not just our spirits that suffer—our physical health deteriorates, too.

Research has shown that people having fewer than four to six satisfying social relationships (with family members, friends, a mate, neighbors, or co-workers) are twice as likely to catch a cold and four times more likely to have a heart attack. This is because loneliness can cause chemical changes in your body, making you more susceptible to illness, says Jeffrey Geller, M.D., a loneliness researcher and director of integrative medicine at the Lawrence Family Practice Residency Program in Lawrence, Massachusetts. A lonely

Mistake to Avoid:

Shape® magazine doesn't include fasting on our list of ways to build spiritual fitness because we believe that to celebrate the richness of the earth's bounty and to keep your mind and body in peak condition, you should enjoy food on a regular basis. Although some religions observe certain holidays by abstaining from food, we do not recommend that you follow this practice on your own.

body will unleash stress hormones (such as cortisol) that suppress the immune system. Good friends are good medicine. If you don't have a strong social connection, not only your soul but your body can suffer:

- You'll have less ability to fight off infection and illnesses such as colds, influenza, cold sores, and other viruses.
- You'll have a higher susceptibility to bacterial infections and perhaps even cancer.
- You're more likely to suffer from depression.
- You're more prone to abuse alcohol and commit suicide.

To nurture your spirit, here's a four-week plan to help you make contact with others in a meaningful way, and how to deepen the connections you already have.

Week One:

Request a small favor. "Most Americans feel very loath to ask favors and to start a reciprocal cycle of helping each other," says Jacqueline Olds, M.D., assistant clinical professor of psychiatry at Harvard Medical School. But if you, say, borrow a cup of milk from your neighbor, she'll be more likely to ask you to water her plants when she's away. Over time, you'll come to rely on each other for other favors, and a friendship may form.

Week Two:

Ask someone in your yoga class (or office or apartment building) out for coffee. If she says she's just too busy, don't assume she's making excuses because she doesn't like you. She really may be too busy to make new friends. Don't take the rejection personally, and move on to someone else. Whatever you do, though, start small. Don't invite someone you've just met to go skiing over the weekend.

Be open to approaching people of other ages, religious backgrounds, races, tastes, interests, and sexual orientations. Not all your buddies need to be 28-year-old, college-educated, single, heterosexual night owls who love Lyle Lovett, Vietnamese food, and sea kayaking just like you. Limiting yourself to a carbon copy of yourself could mean missing out on some great friends.

Week Three:

Take up a hobby. Many women feel lonely because they have no interests to fill their alone time. Do something solo—painting, sewing, swimming laps, playing the piano, learning a foreign language, hiking, photography—so you'll feel more comfortable when you're by yourself. In addition, the more hobbies you have, the more likely you'll be to share common interests with others, and the more attractive you'll be to new friends.

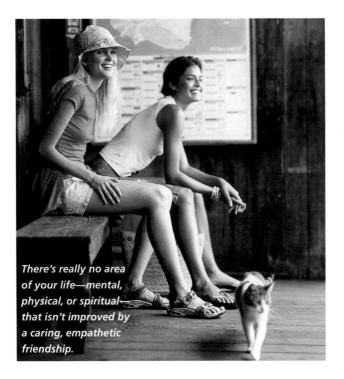

There's really no area of your life—mental, physical, or spiritual—that isn't improved by a caring, empathetic friendship.

Week Four:

Find your "tribe." There's a support group for everyone—new mothers, single parents, overeaters, small-business owners, diabetics—to name but a few. Then there are organizations such as Toastmasters (if you're interested in public speaking) or Mensa (if you have a high I.Q.) or the Sierra Club (if you care about the environment). Check your local bookstore to see if there's a book or poetry club. Take a class where people share your interests.

Join a church, synagogue, or other spiritual community. Being part of a group and observing rituals provides comfort and growth.

7 friends you should have

Here's a list of the seven people we all need (and can be to others) for a healthy, satisfying existence:

1. *The whip cracker.* We all need that tough-love person who pushes us into action. Not sure if you're qualified for a promotion? She's the friend who says, "The job is perfect for you. The moment we hang up, you're making an appointment. Call me back when you've done it."

2. *The mentor.* She's the one you turn to when you have the big questions—what makes for a happy life, what are the keys to success—and who always has the right answers.

3. *The younger friend.* She's the office intern, or the transplant from another city who moved in next door. Make sure she's worthy of your support, then give it to her.

4. *The Mom-away-from-Mom.* She may be the nice older neighbor who brings you soup when you're sick, or the friend's mom who has you over for holiday dinners. Everyone needs a little coddling sometimes.

5. *The translator.* The platonic male friend with sage advice on the male brain. He tells you exactly what your boyfriend means when he says, "I need my space" (start looking for a new boyfriend!).

6. *The comedian.* When you need to de-stress, she's the friend who drags you to a karaoke club or has you rolling with laughter as she relates stories about her dating life.

7. *The best friend.* She's like a caring older sister who watches over you. She's truthful when she thinks someone's bad for you and is the first one you'd call with a 3 A.M. emergency.

volunteering

Volunteering is a two-way street of goodwill. By giving of your time and talents, you can help create the kind of society in which you want to live. In a world filled with intolerance and violence, volunteering is a statement of love, trust, and concern. Whether you choose to get involved to make a difference, to express religious faith, or to give something back for the good fortune you enjoy, you'll reap personal benefits by increasing your sense of belonging and community spirit. Many people have discovered the transformative power of unselfish service and compassion.

The benefits don't stop there. Studies have shown that doing volunteer work results in the release of endorphins, the body's natural opiates, which create a feeling of elation dubbed "helper's high." Health payoffs reported include relief from stress-related conditions such as headaches and backaches as well as overeating, insomnia, and chronic pain. And the most commonly experienced emotional benefit is an increased feeling of self-worth. In order to reap these rewards, you need to engage in direct-contact activities—in other words, writing a check doesn't cut it.

Quick Tip: *If your erratic schedule or family responsibilities keep you from making a regular commitment to volunteer work, try participating in a one-time fund-raising event, such as the Susan G. Komen Race for the Cure or the Revlon Run-Walk. Both are 5K races that raise money to fight breast cancer. Training for the event will give you a great incentive to stick with your fitness plan, too.*

There is one caveat to volunteering. Beware of doing something that might be counterproductive to your well-being. You might find yourself in an extremely demanding or depressing situation in which you seem helpless or out of control. Don't feel weak or guilty if you decide to find some other form of volunteer work to which your temperament and skills are better suited. Similarly, you're likely to become stressed and frustrated if your volunteering endeavors are "success oriented." You'll experience helper's high only when your motivation is to help others.

It's very important in volunteering, perhaps even more so than in other areas of life, that you follow through on your pledge to help. There are people counting on you who could be deeply disappointed if you fail to keep your promises. For that reason, you should take the time to make sure you're not rashly promising something you can't deliver. Here is a four-week plan for helping you decide on the best way to get involved.

Week One:

Make a list of issues that concern you. You can become involved in an infinite number of ways: working with kids, seniors, people with disabilities, or refugees, to name but a few groups of people who often have needs. Then there are issues relating to animal rights, the environment, disaster relief, voter registration, the arts, and more. No matter what your skills or interests, there's some effort going on in your community that could use your help. With volunteering, you can either use the skills you have in fresh creative ways, or learn new ones.

If nothing immediately occurs to you, be mindful when watching TV or reading a magazine. See what catches your attention. Is there a human-interest story that makes you cry, such as animals that have been abused? Some other injustice that enrages you? Talk to friends and relatives. Do you know someone with a medical or social condition that you could fund-raise for? Eventually, you'll hit on topics that engage you.

Week Two:

Find a focus. Now that you've identified broad spheres of interest, you need to work on specifics. Say you wrote down "children." Does that mean babies, grade-schoolers, or high-school kids? You could become involved in areas as diverse as cuddling sick or abandoned infants in a hospital, coaching a girls' soccer team, being a Big Sister, collecting books for a school library, or becoming an advocate for abused kids.

The environment is a popular area of concern. But again, that offers a range of different opportunities. Are you most interested in restoring

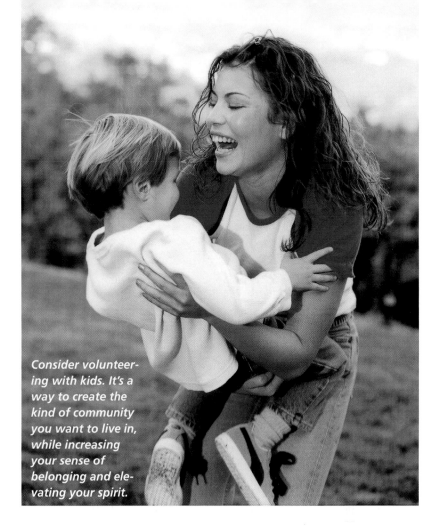

Consider volunteering with kids. It's a way to create the kind of community you want to live in, while increasing your sense of belonging and elevating your spirit.

creeks and rivers, protecting the coastline, safeguarding native plants and wildflowers, or becoming an activist on the subject of air pollution?

As you start to refine your list, you'll see preferences start to emerge. Make a list of priorities.

Week Three:

Decide how much time you can spare. According to a Gallup poll, the most common excuse people give for not volunteering is lack of time. But similar to setting aside time for exercise, you *can* fit in volunteering with good planning and by prioritizing the demands on your time. Start by keeping a log of your daily and weekly activities. Is there an obvious block of time, say, Sunday afternoons, that you could devote to helping a cause? If not, is there some flexible activity such as shopping, that you could rearrange? How about giving up something, such as watching TV, to make room for volunteering? Finally, think about combining it with other activities. For instance, you could make volunteer work a family activity.

There are also some volunteer undertakings that are one-time projects and don't require an ongoing commitment: painting a homeless shelter, cleaning up a beach, or organizing a festival. If you really don't have time in your daily life, you can always plan a volunteer vacation.

"It's a great way to travel while feeling like you're giving something back to the places you're visiting," says 26-year-old *Shape®* reader Suzi Asmus of her experience with Vermont-based Volunteers for Peace. Options might include working in environmental projects such as trail building, organic farming, or building low-income housing and community buildings in countries from Argentina to Zimbabwe.

Mistake to Avoid: *Don't feel that the only religion for you is the one you were born into. There are many meaningful faiths, and the one your family practiced may not always be the most comfortable fit for you. Most religious organizations welcome visitors and newcomers; consider sampling other systems of belief to find a better fit, if that's right for you.*

Week Four:

Start seeking out specific volunteer opportunities. There are numerous ways to find organizations in your community that need you. Places where you might start looking are: your local newspaper; the library; your church, temple, or mosque; your place of employment; a professional association; the Internet; an activist group such as Greenpeace; a charitable foundation such as the March of Dimes or the United Way; your Neighborhood Watch; and/or a hospital.

The main thing is, you need to pick up the phone and ask, "How can I help?"

10 ways to lead a more spiritual life

1. *Connect with others* by choosing live experiences. See plays, not movies; listen to bands instead of CDs; play charades instead of video games.

2. *Make someone else's day.* Throw a surprise party for a friend, or do a favor or an unexpected act of kindness.

3. *Sign up for a charity run/walk.* You'll help a good cause, get outdoors, meet new people, and enjoy a sense of purpose.

4. *Create your own meaningful ceremonies and rituals.* For instance, if you don't want to have a traditional religious holiday, invite friends for a Christmas tree blessing.

5. *Engage your senses.* Make even essential activities more alluring with sensual rituals. Sprinkle your pillow with lavender scent when you launder your sheets, or use luxurious shower gels each morning.

6. *Find an activity that gives you a sense of serenity.* It could be playing the piano or baking bread.

7. *Check out a spiritual custom from another culture* such as feng shui, the Chinese art of placement. It's believed to promote health, positive social relationships, contemplation, and respect for others.

8. *Find out if there's a labyrinth in your neighborhood* (some churches have them). Walking through these medieval contemplation aids is becoming highly popular.

9. *Pause for introspection, perspective, and spirituality.* There are nearly 600 silent retreat centers in the United States and Canada. Contact Retreats International: **www.retreatsintl.org**.

10. *Get a daily dose of "vitamin H,"* better known as humor. Laughing is good for the body and soul.

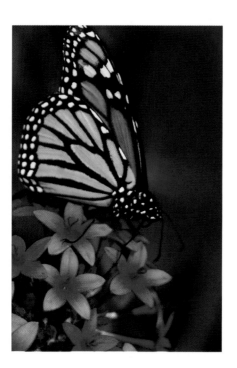

*A connection with nature can bring
serenity to a chaotic, stress-filled life.*

nature

Living in today's world, it's easy to forget that lox from a deli was once a live salmon, or that a glass of water is a precious natural resource from a stream or glacier. Often, the closest we get to nature is watching The Discovery Channel. If that's the case, you may be depriving your spirit and body. Research suggests that a deep connection with nature—or even just *contact* with it—may be an important element of your well-being.

Take fish—they seem to be a natural sedative. "Gaze at an aquarium," says Howard Frumkin, M.D., in the *American Journal of Preventative Medicine*. He found that for patients scheduled to undergo oral surgery, looking at an aquarium for 30 minutes was more relaxing than sitting quietly or looking at a picture of a waterfall.

On the other hand, gazing at landscape photographs seems to sharpen thinking. Research indicates that this is associated with enhanced mental alertness, attention, and cognitive performance.

Treatment in outdoor settings—wilderness therapy—has provided a sense of comfort for many, including bereaved individuals, rape and incest survivors, and cancer patients. Clearly, nature is restorative in all areas of our lives: physical, mental, emotional, and spiritual.

Don't take nature for granted. Develop a sense of awe and wonder when in the natural world. Go out and gaze at the stars, listen to the crashing waves, breathe in the scent of damp earth, celebrate a sunset, or watch the birds in the park.

Although many of us do appreciate nature, few of us enjoy a connection to it in the way that indigenous peoples do. They give thanks to

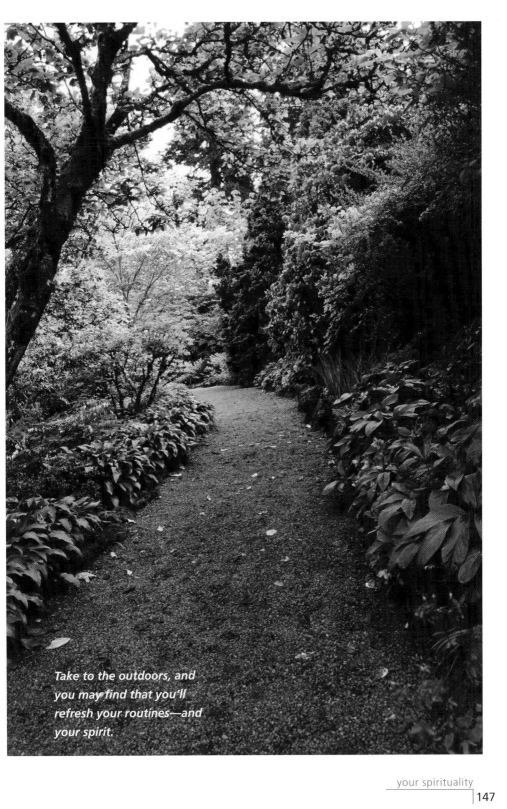

Take to the outdoors, and you may find that you'll refresh your routines—and your spirit.

the natural world and regard it as precious. Our society at best takes its resources for granted, and at worst pollutes or wastes them. One of the ways you can connect with nature is to get involved in preserving the earth's well-being as enthusiastically as you do your own. You can always become a member of an organization such as Greenpeace, the Sierra Club, the Rainforest Action Network, or the Nature Conservancy, all of whom work to slow and repair damage to the natural world. But there's nothing quite like getting your hands dirty to uplift and soothe your spirit. Join or start a local group to save open spaces, plant community gardens and trees, or clean up riverbanks and beaches. (These activities will do double duty, since they fall under the volunteering umbrella, too.)

We have no trouble believing that the daily choices we make about food and exercise have an immediate impact on our well-being. Now consider that our decisions and actions, for better or worse, reach beyond our own bodies to touch the earth as a whole. In time, the earth touches us back.

To get more in touch with nature and reap immense payoffs, follow this plan:

Week One:

Get out of the gym and do part of your exercise in a natural environment, moving and breathing outdoors. Mother Nature is alive and well even in city parks. You could walk, run, cycle, or in-line skate. Do your stretching and yoga outside for a truly soulful experience.

Week Two:

Venture into the wilderness for the weekend. Take advantage of the spectacular national and state parks in North America. Many offer opportunities for hiking, rock climbing, mountain biking, horseback riding, kayaking, or orienteering.

But do you feel that you truly can't get away for a nature break? Then spend a weekend gardening. Getting your hands in the dirt can be soothing and sensual. Even just potting house plants or setting up a kitchen window herb garden works. Besides enriching your spirit, gardening provides health benefits, too. House and garden plants give off oxygen and absorb airborne toxins.

Week Three:

Invite nature indoors. Put a bowl of cut flowers on your desk, or bring a potted lavender plant to work, says Georgia Deutsch, the florist and herbal-wreath teacher at Ojai Valley Inn & Spa in California. "When the flower itself dries out, keep a little dish of the dried petals on your desk. While you're on the phone, play with it, move your fingers around it, and let the aroma come out."

Week Four:

Start planning an outdoor-oriented vacation—there are numerous companies offering sports camps or adventure packages. Ever thought about river rafting, windsurfing, snowboarding, or surviving in the wilderness by your wits? And, of course, there are spas and fitness retreats where you can combine healthy activities with pampering—such as outdoor massages, soothing soaks in hot tubs, and nature-based therapies.

Mistake to Avoid:

Don't be in such a hurry. Our society tends to promote the concept of instant gratification, but in almost every religious tradition, the path to spirituality is a lifelong one.

meditation

Legions of people are finding ways to connect with their spiritual selves in the practice of meditation—a state of deep physical relaxation combined with acute mental alertness.

There are many ways to achieve this state. Almost every religion incorporates meditative practices such as contemplation, repetitive praying, or chanting into their philosophy. Other nonreligious, purely physiological techniques involve sitting and focusing on something that will hold your attention for 5 to 30 minutes, or even longer. This could be a progressive relaxation of your body's muscles, a word, calming music, or an

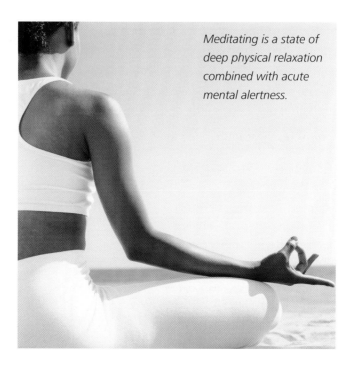

Meditating is a state of deep physical relaxation combined with acute mental alertness.

image. Observing your breath, which naturally tends to become slower and deeper as you relax, is a key part of many techniques.

The benefits of daily practice last far beyond the mere minutes you spend in focus. "Meditation is an instrumental path," says Saki F. Santorelli, Ed.D., director of the Stress Reduction Clinic at the University of Massachusetts Medical School in Worcester and author of *Heal Thy Self*. "Through practicing it, you recognize the possibility of relating to yourself and others in new ways."

In meditation, you also cultivate the art of mindfulness, or paying attention. Being present in the moment can improve the quality of almost everything you do. "Most of the time we're in the past or the future," says Santorelli. "Yet the present is where pleasure and intimacy occur."

As with so much else we've talked about in this chapter; there are health as well as spiritual payoffs to meditating. It has been around for thousands of years as a spiritual practice, but it was only in the 20th century that Western doctors discovered its many physiological benefits. In the 1960s, the Indian guru who popularized Transcendental Meditation (TM), Maharishi Mahesh Yogi, asked Harvard Medical School's Herbert Benson, M.D., to test followers. Benson discovered, and ongoing research has confirmed, that meditation and deep breathing could improve one's health significantly, offsetting the detrimental effects of stress by:

- Decreasing respiratory rate, heart rate, and blood pressure, culminating in what Benson terms "the relaxation response." Physiological effects counter those of the body's stress response (also called the *fight-or-flight response*).

- Relieving muscle tension when combined with progressive relaxation.

- Causing stress hormones in the blood to drop.

- Boosting immunity.

- Being more restful than a nap: Meditation causes oxygen consumption (a measure of how hard the body is working) to drop more than it does while you sleep.

There are many reasons to think you can't meditate—you're too busy, too undisciplined, or distracted—but meditation is so diverse that there *is* a form of it for you. In fact, there's no wrong way to meditate. Experiment with different techniques until you find one that you like, then adapt it to suit your own personality—because that's the one that will encourage you to stick with the practice.

As with anything that's truly worth doing, you need to be motivated. You can't find time to practice meditation—you have to *make* it. Try going to bed a half hour earlier so you can get up earlier to meditate, or closing your office door and holding all calls for 15 minutes. Apart from formal meditation, you have many more hours a day that offer opportunities to snatch short moments of informal meditation time. While walking between appointments, taking a shower, or before falling asleep, take a few conscious breaths and savor the sensory pleasures of the moment. Mindfulness goes far beyond any one technique. In its many forms, meditation is simply about experiencing yourself. To reap the benefits of meditation, you have to practice regularly. Here's a program to help you get into the habit.

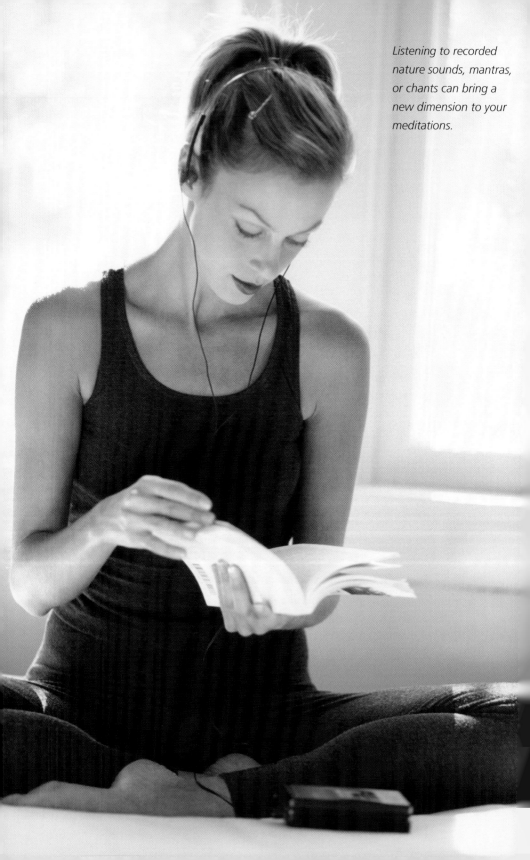

Listening to recorded nature sounds, mantras, or chants can bring a new dimension to your meditations.

Week One:

To get a taste of the meditative experience, try this simple exercise every day this week:

1. Sit quietly in a comfortable position and close your eyes. Deeply relax all your muscles, beginning at your feet and progressing up to your face. Keep them relaxed.

2. Breathe through your nose. Become aware of each inhalation and exhalation, but don't force deep breaths. As you breathe out, silently say the word *one*. Breathe easily and naturally, and continue for 10 to 20 minutes.

3. When your thoughts inevitably wander, gently direct your attention back to breathing and repeating "one."

Week Two:

Experiment with different forms. Meditation is traditionally associated with a sitting position, but if you can barely keep still, you might enjoy a Buddhist walking meditation. Walk slowly, paying attention to the feel of your feet touching the ground and gazing at a spot a few steps ahead of you.

If you prefer noise to silence, play a CD of environmental sounds to help you focus. Or try chanting. You can chant during meditation by repeating a simple mantra, such as "ohm" or "ahh," or "peace." There are also chanting CDs that you can sing along to. Spring Hill Music has a whole catalog of sacred chant music. A good sampler is *Chant: Spirit in Sound,* which has 25 chants from cultures as diverse as the Apache and Sufi traditions.

You can even meditate while you're working out. Next time you're on the treadmill or the stair machine, take off your headphones and save the reading material for later. Instead of trying to ward off boredom or focusing on results, be present with what's going on in your body: your breath, the flexing of your muscles, and the intensity of a stretch.

Quick Tip: *If writing in a traditional diary-style journal makes you uncomfortable, invent an imaginary pen pal and write an e-mail to her every day, sharing your feelings. You may find that you're more relaxed using the informal style of e-mail, and that your thoughts flow more naturally than when you're writing with pen and paper. Then you can e-mail the message to yourself or just store it unsent in a personal file.*

Week Three:

Rent or buy some guided audio or video meditations. Many prominent scholars and teachers of the discipline have made recordings that are very useful for helping you concentrate. Some are basic "how-to" guides. Others are purely physical exercises such as breathing or body relaxation meditations. One we recommend is *Meditations for Relaxation and Stress Reduction* by Joan Borysenko, Ph.D. Many are linked to ancient religious or spiritual traditions. Quite a few audio tapes have three or four different techniques for you to try. Daniel Goleman, Ph.D., compiles four—breath, body scan, walking, and mindfulness meditations—on *The Art of Meditation*. This is a great way to help you find the best way for *you* to tap in to a deeper understanding of yourself and your world. A browse around a bookstore or **Amazon.com** will reap a world of new ideas.

Week Four:

Try taking a meditation group or class. Meditating in the company of others can be a profoundly moving experience. It's not difficult these days to find a group. In Los Angeles, for example, where *Shape*® magazine is based, the Yellow Pages actually has listings for "Meditation Instruction." Look for a Buddhist temple, as they often hold sessions that are open to the public, and some even provide training. Your doctor or local hospital might be able to direct you toward a group, since so many medical institutions now employ meditation as a stress-reducing method.

Even if you feel that you prefer meditation to be a solo endeavor, it's still worth trying the group experience once.

journaling

If you've ever poured out your feelings onto the printed page, you know how much better it can make you feel.

Experts in the field of "journaling," as it's known, say that writing can help with just about anything that causes you spirit-sapping stress and anxiety.

"A journal is like your close friend; you can say anything to it," says Jon Progoff, director of Dialogue House Associates, an organization in New York City that gives intensive journal workshops. "Through the process of writing, there's healing, there's awareness, and there's growth."

But lately, science is also standing behind the pen and paper as a way to heal both spiritually and physically. Journal writing gained a scientific thumbs-up in a published study of about 112 patients with asthma or rheumatoid arthritis—two chronic, debilitating diseases. Some of the patients wrote about the most stressful event in their lives, and others wrote about emotionally neutral topics such as their daily plans. When the study ended after four months, the writers who faced the skeletons in their emotional closets were healthier: Asthma patients showed a 19 percent improvement in lung function, and rheumatoid arthritis sufferers showed a 28 percent drop in the severity of their symptoms.

Researchers aren't quite sure why writing helps, but the evidence does strongly suggest that venting on paper about painful events can reduce stress. This is important because stress can depress your immune system, raise your blood pressure, and skew your hormonal functions. Research conducted by James W. Pennebaker, Ph.D., professor of psychology at the University of Texas at Austin, has shown that people who write about traumatic events do improve their lives: students do better in class; and the unemployed are more likely to find jobs. These individuals are even able to be better friends, and we already know the importance of close attachments to others.

Furthermore, writing in a journal helps you uncover solutions and strengths that may be lying buried within you. Like meditation, journal writing allows your mind to focus quietly and completely on accepting something painful from your past or figuring out how best to deal with a problem. Often we don't know what we know until we see it in black and white.

Here are some pointers for starting to journal:

Week One:

Every day, set aside 15 to 20 minutes to write in your journal. Pick a quiet, undisturbed place. (On the other hand, some people like to write in a coffee shop with a bottomless cup for inspiration.) Don't worry about handwriting, grammar, or spelling.

Explore what you're feeling. If you've been fired, for instance, write about your fears ("What if I can't get another job?"), connections to your childhood ("My father was unemployed a lot and we never had enough money"), and your future ("I want to live in a smaller town").

Week Two:

Try different writing styles. Write a speech to the boyfriend who dumped you, a dialogue between your sedentary, overweight self and the healthier self you want to be, or letters of forgiveness. These techniques can help you let go of the blame and anger that blocks unconditional love and spirituality.

Week Three:

Of course, you won't always have unhappy or disturbing events to write about. This week, switch to creating a gratitude journal. Each day, make a list of ten things for which you're thankful. Expressing gratitude opens you up to more positive experiences.

Week Four:

Write your own credo (beginning "I believe . . .") to examine what your heart and soul are trying to tell you. It will help you determine what you believe in and clarify your values. Each day, write down some suggestions on how you could put these concepts into action in your life.

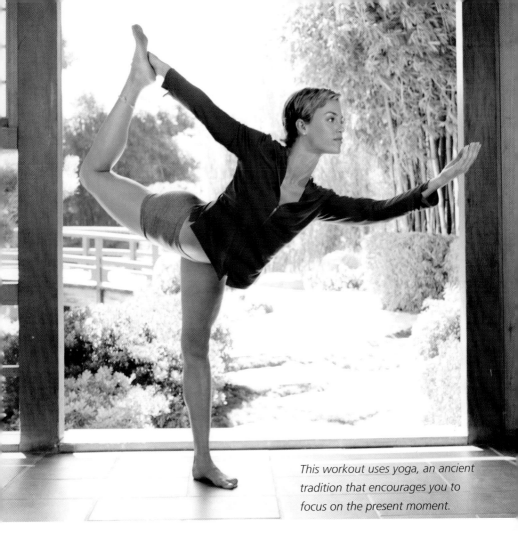

This workout uses yoga, an ancient tradition that encourages you to focus on the present moment.

the mindful exercise workout

The last few years have seen a change in the types of classes and activities offered by gyms. They're beginning to focus on soothing the spirit as well as energizing the body. Think waterfalls, incense, and New Age music . . . instead of TV sets and blaring rock music. Some health clubs are offering stretch classes lit by aromatherapy candles, and Zen-inspired classes featuring live instrumental music. They're evidently catching on that fitness includes the entire package.

However, you don't have to join a health club to reap the benefits of these activities. Almost any activity can be better for body and soul if you

Quick Tip: *Confused about the difference between yoga, tai chi, and qi gong, and not sure which is right for you? All three share meditative qualities and are good for quieting the mind. Qi gong is the ancient Chinese practice from which the martial art of tai chi evolved, so the two are similar in that they focus on directing energy through the body and are practiced with slow concentration while standing. Yoga, which originated in India, involves a series of stretching and twisting postures and is more physically demanding. It has many disciplines, including the fast-paced Ashtanga form.*

do it mindfully, but some popular forms of exercise such as yoga, tai chi, and qi gong are actually rooted in spiritual traditions. The increased interest in them parallels the general surge in spiritual questing in our society.

The most widespread of these practices, of course, is yoga. In the last ten years, millions of Americans have realized what an incredible, all-purpose exercise it is. Deep, energizing breaths combined with fluid movement and challenging poses yield tremendous physical benefits: increased flexibility, strength, and muscle tone. Some forms, such as Ashtanga, increase cardiovascular fitness, too.

Yoga is also a moving meditation that helps you cultivate energy, focus on the moment, calm your mind, and tap in to your soul. In fact, any exercise can become mindful when you shut out the outside world and tune in to your body, paying attention to your breathing, the working of your muscles, and the associated sensations.

Yoga expert Rodney Yee created the sequence of moves illustrated, which are demonstrated by actress Jennifer Grant, who practices four times a week. According to Yee, the key is focus: As you hold each pose, observe how your body is responding. Are you clenching your face? Holding your breath? If so, try to free your body of the unnecessary tension. You may feel like you're not working as hard at first, but ultimately your mindfulness will pay off.

the plan

To get started in yoga, do each of the following moves in sequence at least three times a week. Do an equal number of sequences, alternating sides each time you perform one-sided moves such as Warrior I, Warrior II, and Side Plank. Move smoothly between each posture.

The first week, hold each move for two or three breath inhalation/exhalation cycles. Work up to holding first for 30 seconds, then progressing to two minutes after four weeks of practice. As you perform the moves, pay attention to your breathing: When you inhale, push your belly out slightly and expand your ribs. When you exhale, let your belly fall back to its natural position. Breathe through your nose, not your mouth. Finish this sequence by resting in *sayasana,* lying on your back, arms by your sides, a few inches away from your body with your palms up. Your legs should be relaxed and slightly open. Focus on breathing slowly and evenly.

As you slowly move from one into the next, concentrate on maintaining your alignment and not holding your breath. Exhale as you move into each pose, and then inhale and breathe deeply as you hold and relax.

Warm up with some easy cardio—perhaps a walk outside—taking time to notice your surroundings. Cool down at the end by gently stretching all the major muscles. Hold each stretch position 15 to 30 seconds, focusing on your breathing.

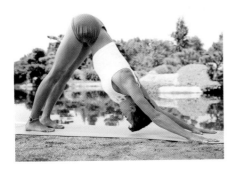

1. Downward-Facing Dog.
Begin on all fours with your toes turned under and hands flat on the ground, just in front of your shoulders. Your head, neck, back, and hips should form a straight line. Inhale, pressing hands into the ground. As you exhale, straighten legs and lift hips up so your whole body makes a triangle with the ground as the base. Your weight should be distributed evenly between your hands and feet. Extend your spine by pressing hands down and thighs back, pulling your hips up, reaching heels toward the ground as much as possible. Concentrate on breathing as you hold this position for 30 seconds.

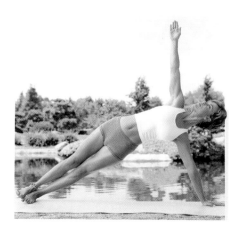

2. Side-Arm Balance. *From Downward-Facing Dog, inhale and rotate your torso to the right, lowering left hip and lifting right hip up and back until you're supported on your left hand and the outside of your left foot (from head to feet, your body forms a straight line that points diagonally toward the ground). Stack right foot on top of left, keeping both legs straight, so ankle bones are together (as if you're standing). Keeping left arm straight and slightly in front of left shoulder, raise right arm in the air until it's perpendicular to your torso (so you form a cross with your body). Keep abs contracted, pelvis stable, and back in a neutral position; hold for 15 seconds. (Modification: Bend left leg so knee is on the ground.) Rotate whole body toward the ground, place left hand on ground, and go back into Downward-Facing Dog.*

Repeat Side-Arm Balance on opposite side; then go back into another Downward-Facing Dog before continuing on to next move.

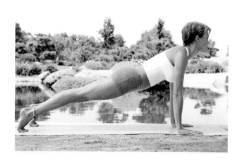

3. Plank Pose. *From Downward-Facing Dog, keeping your arms and legs straight, drop your hips until your head, hips, and legs form a straight line (a full push-up position). Pushing slightly from your toes, shift body weight a little forward. Breathing deeply, hold for 10 seconds.*

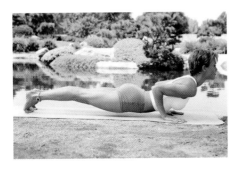

4. Bent-Arm Plank. *From Plank Pose, keep elbows close to your sides as you bend your arms and lower your body (keeping it straight) toward the ground until your elbows are as close to even with your shoulders (90 degrees) as possible. Looking forward, keep chest open and shoulder blades down. Breathe evenly and hold for 5 seconds. Straighten arms and hold for ten seconds in Plank Pose. Lift hips up to Downward-Facing Dog.*

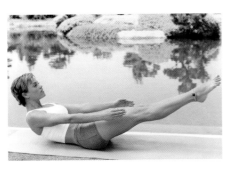

5. Half Boat. *From Downward-Facing Dog, bring your legs forward to a cross-legged sitting position; then lie on your back, legs extended. Bend knees in toward chest and put hand on the back of your thighs, shins parallel to the ground. Holding this position, straighten knees to extend legs in front of you so feet are at eye level; hold for 5 seconds. Pull your body up a bit more, extend arms toward feet, and breathe evenly as you hold for 5 seconds. Repeat this pose one to three times.*

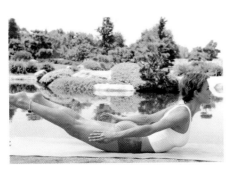

6. Locust. *From Half Boat, lower and roll over so you're lying flat on your belly, legs extended, and arms alongside your body, palms and forehead down. Contract buttocks, anchoring hips firmly on the ground. Squeezing shoulder blades together, lift head and chest up and forward off the ground while reaching arms behind you; at the same time, lift legs off the ground. At the top position, you'll balance on lower belly and hips (with both ends of your body pulling away from each other). Lower slowly, come up to all fours, turning toes under; and then lift hips upward into Downward-Facing Dog.*

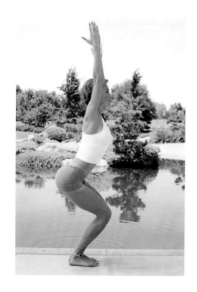

7. Power Pose. From Downward-Facing Dog, step forward with your right foot through your arms and into a lunge. Then bring your left foot forward next to the right (slightly apart is okay for balance), knees bent so thighs are close to parallel to the ground (as if you're sitting in a chair). Raise arms overhead, looking forward and curving spine naturally. Draw abs in toward spine. Breathe evenly as you hold for at least 30–45 seconds.

8. Forward Bend. From Power Pose, bend forward from your hips (supporting yourself with hands on thighs, if necessary), folding your upper body over your thighs until your hands touch the ground. Hang relaxed for 45–60 seconds, knees straight or bent, depending on your comfort level.

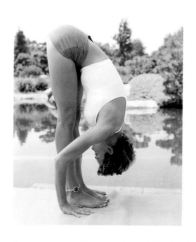

9. Relaxation Pose (not shown). From Forward Bend, kneel on the ground. Then lie down on your back, legs comfortably separated; let feet fall open. Relax arms by sides, palms up, head straight, and eyes closed. Breathe normally, and mentally scan your body, letting go of any tensions you're holding. Continue to breathe as you become completely relaxed, both physically and mentally. Stay in this position for at least 5 minutes before you return to your day.

the program in action

Gloria Zuroff of Utah was a *Shape*® Success Stories subject. When she first appeared in the magazine, she'd gained 45 pounds after a lifelong battle with anorexia. She ate a healthful diet and ran five to six miles, weight trained, and stair climbed every other day. A few years later, she joined three other Success Stories alumnae at Canyon Ranch Spa in Arizona for a makeover. All had overcome some sort of obstacle and had an understanding of what the others had been through. Connecting instantly, they even named themselves the "*Shape*® Sisters."

At Canyon Ranch, experts advised Gloria to include yoga, stretching, or a relaxation activity in her workout schedule. At first she wondered how she would benefit from yoga—but she found that it kept her mind centered at her high-stress job as a hospital lab director and helped her through a divorce. She finally felt that she was in control of her well-being, and as time went by, her bond with her *Shape*® Sisters grew stronger.

Then Gloria fell at work, injuring her back. Her doctor's diagnosis: a herniated disc, which required surgery. "I couldn't work out during the weeks after the surgery, I was in so much pain," she recalls. Her doctor also recommended yoga and stretching. Convinced she needed to do something to begin her recovery, she returned to her yoga practice and gradually regained flexibility. Gloria also hired a trainer who helped her design a weight-training program to rebuild her strength. Six months later, she felt strong and healthy again. During her recovery, she stayed in close contact with her *Shape*® Sisters.

Totally well today, Gloria believes that yoga techniques have helped her stay in touch with her body and heal faster. And the support of her *Shape*® Sisters had a hand in it, too. "They called, sent letters, and helped keep my spirits up."

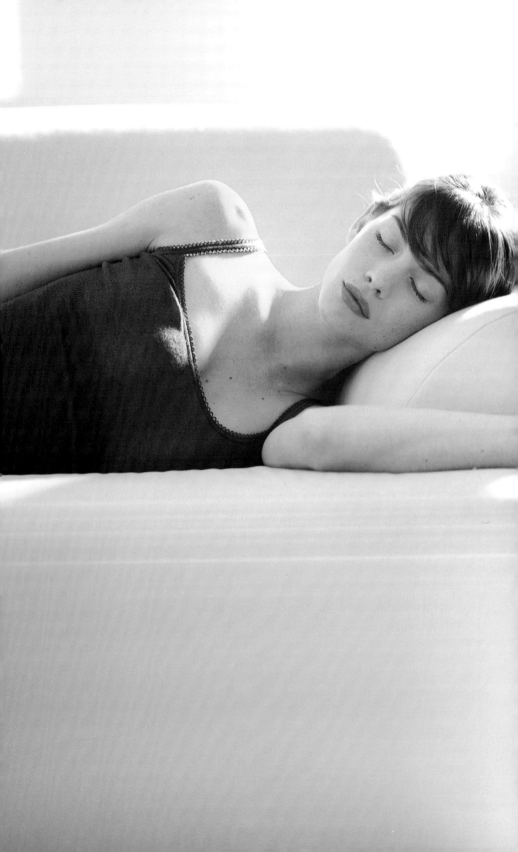

chapter four
your rest

Quick Tip: *Snagging a 15- to 20-minute nap between 1 and 4 P.M. can improve your alertness, sharpen your memory, and help reduce fatigue. Can't fit in a siesta? Try reserving this lull in alertness for less mentally demanding activities.*

what you'll learn

Adequate sleep, rest, and renewel are vital components of overall physical, mental, and emotional health. In fact, sleep may be the missing link in your fitness program.

Using the information in this chapter, you'll:

- learn how to get the sleep you need
- enhance the quality of your sleep
- help your weight maintenance
- get restorative downtime
- make the most of your vacations
- improve your workouts by giving yourself necessary rest and recovery

how you'll do it

You've seen the word *work* many times in this book already, as in "work out," "working at sticking to your healthy eating plan," and "volunteer work," and there's more to come in future chapters. But for a little while, work takes a vacation. Now is the time to look at the other, and equally important, side of the coin—sleep and its kin: rest, recovery, and renewel. Unfortunately, all three are sadly lacking in many of our lives, and it's important to turn that around for optimal health.

what's the story with sleep?

In the days before humankind began living under artificial lighting, things used to be simple: We'd go to sleep when the world turned too cool and too dark for us to work or play. We'd wake up naturally when the sun came up, providing us with light to see by and warmth for our bodies. But now that we use technology to manipulate our environment, enjoy nightlife, work graveyard shifts, and travel across times zones, most of us aren't getting all the nocturnal nourishment we need.

Burning the midnight oil cramming for an exam or working toward a promotion? Finding that your sleep is being disrupted because there's a new baby in the house? Partying until all hours because you "only live once"? You may think it's no big deal—after all, you're young and healthy. But you won't be for long if you keep up that lifestyle. It may sound dramatic, but researchers are finding that losing sleep can be as detrimental to your mind and body as not exercising or eating poorly. Yet many of us skimp on rest, either by choice or because we're unable to sleep.

"There are no shortcuts for sleep, but that doesn't stop people from trying to constrain the amount of time they spend on it," says Martin Moore-Ede, M.D., a Harvard Medical School physiology professor and CEO of Circadian Technologies, a Boston fatigue consulting firm.

Not only can insufficient sleep make us feel groggy and moody, but it also negatively affects our concentration abilities, reduces creativity, promotes memory loss, contributes to conditions such as diabetes and hypertension, and leaves us less able to tolerate stress. Sleep deprivation also damages our immune system, which we constantly challenge all day in our

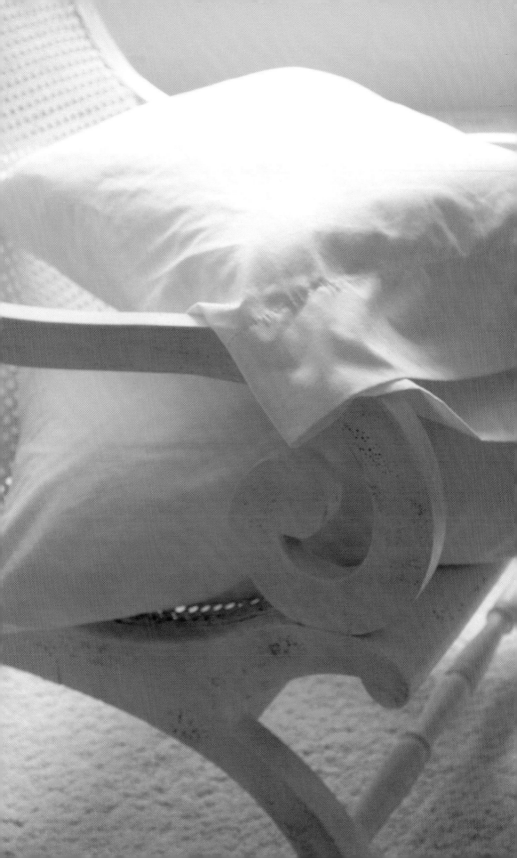

encounters with germs, smog, smoke, and other elements that attack our bodies. Slumber is really the only opportunity for the immune system to rejuvenate itself, since when we don't sleep for a sufficient number of hours, it can't repair itself as well.

Habitually getting less sleep than we need can even accelerate the aging process. A University of Chicago study found that when healthy men ages 17 to 28 were restricted to four hours of sleep for six nights in a row, their blood pressure, blood sugar, and memory loss increased to levels usually associated with 60-year-olds. (Fortunately, after a few nights of 12-hour slumbers, they were able to turn back the clock.)

Sleeplessness can also be dangerous: Recent research shows that there are more drowsy drivers on the road than drunken drivers, and they're more likely than people driving under the influence to make potentially fatal mistakes, such as falling asleep at the wheel. Even if you don't succumb to sleep, fatigue slows your reaction time in critical situations. The bottom line is that we need sleep, and fighting to keep ourselves awake when our bodies crave it can have detrimental effects on our well-being.

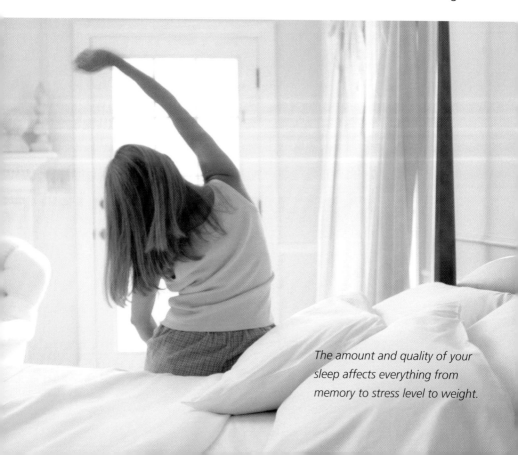

The amount and quality of your sleep affects everything from memory to stress level to weight.

do you have a sleep disorder?

Sometimes, not being able to sleep is indicative of a deeper problem. Take our quiz to see if you need to consult a doctor.

YES   NO

___ ___ 1. Even after eight hours of sleep, I feel tired when the alarm goes off.

___ ___ 2. I'm often stiff and achy when I wake up.

___ ___ 3. I frequently have disturbing dreams.

___ ___ 4. I sometimes wake up gasping for breath.

___ ___ 5. My partner says that I snore.

___ ___ 6. My partner's snoring keeps me awake.

___ ___ 7. My daytime sleepiness has caused me to have accidents.

___ ___ 8. I'm cranky from fatigue almost every day.

___ ___ 9. Heartburn keeps me awake.

___ ___ 10. I can't sleep even when I'm exhausted.

SCORING

If you answered yes to two or more of these questions, you should discuss your sleep problems with a health-care professional. They might want to check you out for a host of conditions including anemia, hypothyroidism, bruxism (teeth grinding), side effects from drugs such as antidepressants or cold medicines, sleep apnea (episodes of interrupted breathing), a poor diet, or stress. To find a sleep-disorder specialist, contact the American Academy of Sleep Medicine at (708) 492-0930 or **www.aasmnet.org/listing.htm**.

the sleep/weight connection

Not yet convinced that you need to get enough shut-eye? Then consider this: If you don't get plenty of sleep, your workouts may be less effective and you're likely to store more fat. It has to do with a stress-associated hormone called *cortisol.*

When you don't get sufficient sleep, your body produces more cortisol, which is largely responsible for waking you up in the morning. When you *are* getting adequate sleep, cortisol levels are usually at their highest at around 5 to 6 A.M. and begin a slow decline throughout the day. By the time you tumble into bed, you're feeling more relaxed and ready for sleep.

When you're not getting enough sleep, the body produces more cortisol. Although you may be able to fall asleep, your cortisol-tinged slumber won't be as restful or beneficial to the body's repair. "Cortisol depletes the muscles by causing cellular breakdown," says Pamela Peeke, M.D., M.P.H., author of *Fight Fat After Forty.* "If your cortisol is high while you're trying to sleep, your muscles are weaker, and any muscle-building exercises you do during your workouts could be less effective."

Higher levels of cortisol also turn on a fat-storing enzyme to increase fat storage. And while cortisol may initially decrease appetite, there's a rebound increase in appetite that follows. Fatigue makes us feel like we're low on fuel, and one of the most common antidotes we use to combat that drained feeling is to eat when we're not really hungry. Furthermore, elevated cortisol may affect junk-food cravings, causing nighttime munchfests of carbs and fatty foods.

> **Quick Tip:** *Tryptophan, a sleep-promoting amino acid, is found in dairy products, fish, poultry, pumpkins, and sunflower seeds. Nutritionists say that carbohydrates help tryptophan cross into the brain. So try having a small bowl of cereal and low-fat milk, or some nonfat yogurt and a cracker before bedtime.*

Another unhealthful behavior related to sleep deprivation is turning to caffeine to give you an energy boost after a bad night's sleep. While one or two cups of coffee or soda a day haven't been proven to have long-term detrimental effects, many people tend to consume more than that when they're feeling exhausted. But the caffeine jolt lasts only so long before we plunge back into our sleepy state. "Using caffeine when you're tired is ignoring what your body is telling you. It's like being cold and refusing to put on a sweater," says Cynthia Sass, R.D., a dietitian at the University of South Florida in Tampa. She adds, "Caffeine is a false energy source. All it does is stimulate the nervous system."

What's more, some people are much more sensitive to caffeine than others. "Some of my clients tell me that they can drink a strong cup of coffee right before bedtime and have no difficulty falling asleep. Others can't tolerate any caffeine without it affecting their ability to fall asleep," says Sass. Caffeine is more likely to interfere with sleep when it's taken by someone who rarely has it, or someone with a morning latte habit who's unaccustomed to drinking caffeine later in the day. (For instance, if you normally don't drink coffee after noon, and then you have a post-dinner espresso one evening, you may have trouble sleeping that night.) Furthermore, caffeine is a diuretic, contributing to dehydration, which in turn can interrupt your sleep when thirst awakens you during the night. "Taking a short catnap and making sure you're adequately hydrated are much more effective ways to boost energy than grabbing a caffeinated drink," say Sass.

tossing (and turning) hormones into the mix

Just being a woman may account for your not getting enough sleep. Do you have occasional trouble sleeping? If your restless nights last just a few days, but then return in about four weeks, you probably have insomnia related to menstruation. The National Sleep Foundation in Washington, D.C., polled 1,000 women and found that 36 percent of them had period-related sleep problems.

Lately, more attention is being focused on the effects of hormones such as estrogen and progesterone on sleep cycles. Sleep researcher Martin Moore-Ede, M.D., says that in general, women report more trouble sleeping than men do. Although this may be due to sociological factors, fluctuating levels of hormones are at least partially responsible for the quality of sleep women get.

Mistake to Avoid: *Don't dismiss snoring as merely an annoyance. Research reveals that about 31 percent of women snore a few nights a week, and the most common cause is being overweight—providing another good reason to get in shape. Snoring can also be a symptom of sleep apnea, a potentially serious condition in which you periodically stop breathing during the night.*

"As hormone levels rise and fall, they affect a woman's ability to sleep," says Joyce Walsleben, Ph.D., director of the New York University Sleep Disorders Center in Manhattan. "Some women are more sensitive to those fluctuations than others."

Researchers believe that the hormone progesterone is the cause. When levels are high, women sleep well; when levels fall, sleep can be elusive. About a week before your period, your progesterone level peaks. Then over the next few days, it falls rapidly. The uterine wall begins to break down, and PMS symptoms, including sleeplessness, kick in.

PMS-related sleep problems vary. Some women report trouble falling asleep; others can't stay asleep; still others don't feel refreshed when they wake up in the morning. Walsleben says that a healthy sleeper spends 10 to 15 percent of her sleep time in deep sleep, but women with PMS spend only about 5 percent in deep sleep, causing that morning grogginess.

Minimizing stress and exercising regularly can reduce symptoms such as bloating, irritability, and cramps, which can also cause insomnia. Also, get your full quota of sleep when you can, because exhaustion can intensify

fight fatigue with fitness

If you got a good night's sleep but are exhausted after a draining day at work, it's probably your mind, not your body, that's tired. And although exercise taxes your muscles and expends calories, it may be just what you need to fight your fatigue. "Exercise has a relaxing yet energizing effect that can play a powerful role in relieving feelings of fatigue and exhaustion," says Jack Raglin, Ph.D., an exercise psychologist in the department of kinesiology at Indiana University in Bloomington.

Science is proving exercise to be such an effective energizer that some doctors are using it to combat illnesses such as depression and chronic fatigue. Experts cite a host of physiological and neurological mechanisms that work together to rev up your mind and body. Among them are increased circulation, deep breathing that whisks energizing oxygen to your muscles, and the release of "feel good" neurochemicals. Exercising also relieves stress, which is so tiring to lug around.

Walking, swimming, or an energy-boosting discipline such as tai chi or qi gong are great pick-me-ups. Just remember not to do them too close to bedtime.

PMS symptoms. "Women tend to eat more when they're tired from PMS, instead of sleeping, which is what they actually need," says Peeke.

Fluctuating hormones can also be responsible for poor sleep during various stages of pregnancy and again during perimenopause. As Peeke explains, perimenopause is like long, drawn-out PMS. It's the constant waxing and waning of estrogen and progesterone that causes the body's thermometer to rise, sometimes very quickly. Known as hot flashes, these hormonal changes can make you feel uncomfortable and stressed, and that invites an extra dose of cortisol into your system. Thanks to that additional cortisol, you begin the cycle of inadequate or nonrestorative sleep.

10 ways to get a good night's sleep

1. *Get regular exposure to daylight, especially in the afternoon.* (Research shows that night-shift workers can improve daytime sleep by working under bright lights.)

2. *Start to reduce light around the house for a while before bedtime.* Use dimmer switches, or turn off some lamps.

3. *Don't allow yourself to nod off on the sofa.* When you become drowsy, go to bed.

4. *Use your bedroom only to sleep and have sex.* Don't make it a satellite office, study hall, or entertainment center.

5. *When you can't sleep, try relaxing imagery and thoughts,* as well as slow, deep-breathing techniques.

6. *If you haven't dropped off within about 20 minutes, get up and read,* or engage in some other quiet activity. Go back to bed when you get sleepy.

7. *Put the alarm clock out of sight.* Clock watching doesn't help you sleep and may even keep you awake.

8. *Sleep specialists recommend lying on your back or your side,* not your stomach.

9. *Get Fido and Fluffy their own comfy beds.* In a study conducted by the Mayo Clinic, half the people surveyed had their sleep disturbed by pets.

10. *Only take over-the-counter sleep aids as an occasional emergency measure.* You can build up a tolerance to them very quickly. If you find yourself relying on them, see your doctor.

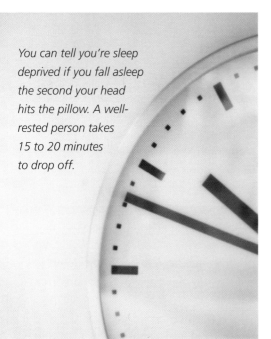

You can tell you're sleep deprived if you fall asleep the second your head hits the pillow. A well-rested person takes 15 to 20 minutes to drop off.

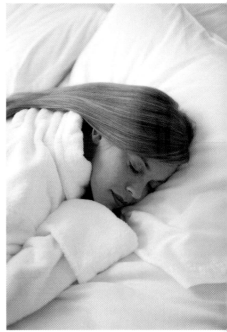

how much is enough?

If you aren't getting adequate sleep, you're not alone. According to the National Sleep Foundation, 40 percent of Americans say they feel so tired during the day that it interferes with their activities. So exactly how much sleep do you need? As a general rule, most adults require one hour of sleep for every two they're awake, hence the eight-hour benchmark used by many sleep experts. Yet, according to Cornell University psychology professor James B. Maas, Ph.D., author of *Power Sleep,* "For peak performance, 8 hours of sleep is not the ideal. It's 9 hours and 25 minutes." American women on average get only about 6 hours and 10 minutes of sleep. That is three hours less than she needs through age 25 (to accommodate effects of puberty and post-puberty hormones) and nearly two hours less than she needs after age 25, says Maas.

When we get less sleep than we need, our bodies start to build what researchers call "sleep debt." Here's how the formula works: If you get only six hours sleep each day, you tack two hours onto your debt. Two nights' worth of debt, or four hours, makes you more irritable. Five days' worth of deprivation—ten hours less than you need, which is more than an entire night's sleep—can increase the chance of health problems such as coughs and colds. Additional sleep debt increases your risk of being involved in an accident, whether it's as inconsequential as bumping your shin on the coffee table or as serious as wrecking your car on the highway.

If you're among those who believe that they can compensate for their sleep debt with naps or by sleeping late on the weekend, note that even the laziest Sunday morning in bed won't make up for a bad week of rest. While making up as much snoozing as you can does help somewhat (and your make-up sleep is usually deeper, more restorative sleep, so you needn't match your deficit hour for hour), chances are that your performance during the week still isn't optimal. Plus, sleeping in on weekends can disrupt your sleep cycle later in the week. You're better off going to bed and waking up at a set time every day, even on your days off from work. Allowing your sleep debt to accumulate week after week eventually means that you can't completely rid yourself of it.

By not allowing sleep to clean up the cellular debris from your day and let new cells generate, your body starts to exhibit the effects of burnout. Think of your body as an office building, suggests Pamela Peeke, M.D. Housecleaning arrives at night to remove the garbage and straighten everything up for the next day. If a group of executives works all night long, when is the cleaning crew going to have a chance to do its job? The building will still be in disarray the next day, but ready or not, that company's got to carry on business as usual. And if those executives insist on continually working late into the night, there's no way housecleaning will ever catch up. The deterioration of the building—inevitable without periodic repairs—will simply accelerate. While we often skimp on sleep so we can indulge in some "you only live once" late-night reveling, maintaining a low-sleep lifestyle can actually hasten the end of youth.

"We live in a 24/7 world, and sleep consumes time, one of life's most precious commodities," says Moore-Ede. But, he adds, "we cannot function or survive without sleep. It's one of the fundamental requirements of life, just like food and water."

So it's imperative in this fast-paced world that we get the rest our bodies truly need. The first step is the acknowledgment that you *need* it. Then the next time you consider staying up for that late-night movie, maybe you'll think twice.

everything you need to know about insomnia (but were too tired to ask)

Okay, you're trying to get an adequate amount of sleep, but it simply eludes you. You know the feeling: You lie in bed trying to will yourself to nod off, watching the clock tick closer to dawn. Nearly all adults will experience insomnia during their lifetime. It can be transient (last just a few days), intermittent (recurring from time to time), or chronic (lasting for more than a month and occurring on most nights).

Stress, depression, and anxiety play the biggest roles in keeping you up nights. Dealing with these emotions (there's more about that in the next chapter) is the first step to ensuring a good night's sleep. But there are other culprits that tend to keep you awake. Common insomnia patterns and causes are:

- *You can't fall sleep.* You find it difficult to drop off within 30 minutes of going to bed. Strenuous exercise, heavy meals that leave you with indigestion, and alcohol or caffeine too close to bedtime are common causes. Other sleep preventers are television, radio, and stimulating music in the bedroom.

- *You wake up in the middle of the night, sometimes more than once.* Sleep robbers such as PMS, menstrual cramps, the need to urinate, pregnancy, new motherhood, and a

> **Mistake to Avoid:**
>
> *Don't rely on TV to lull you to sleep. Television programs can stimulate your alertness. Plus, the flickering light keeps you awake. Worse, if you do fall asleep with the TV on, the light will make your sleep shallow and unsatisfactory.*

snoring mate or disruptive pet can awaken you throughout the night. You also could have a medical condition such as a breathing disorder, arthritis, or restless-legs syndrome (which triggers an involuntary "crawling" sensation).

- *You wake up too early.* Your eyes fly wide open at least 90 minutes before the alarm goes off and you can't go back to sleep. Perhaps your neighborhood is noisy, your room is too light, or you're too hot or cold. Maybe you simply went to bed early and have had enough sleep.

If you're experiencing any of these patterns, follow our four-week plan for getting a good night's sleep.

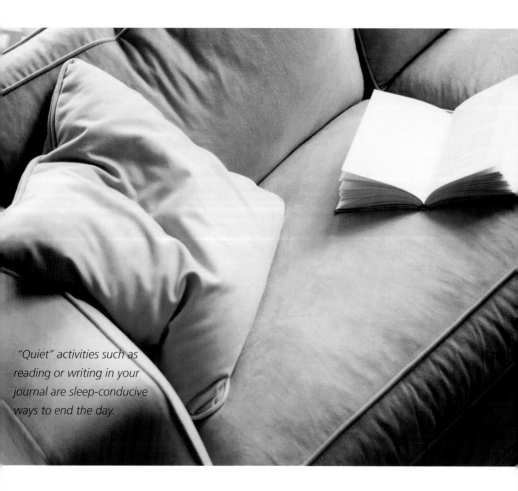

"Quiet" activities such as reading or writing in your journal are sleep-conducive ways to end the day.

Week One:

Start keeping a sleep journal. Write down what time you got to bed, how long you think it took you to fall asleep, how many times you woke up during the night, and what time you awoke in the morning. Also note how you felt during the day. Did you get up feeling refreshed? Did you become tired or sleepy in the afternoon? If so, what time? At the end of the week, you should have a good idea of your sleep patterns.

Week Two:

Keep going with your sleep journal, but now begin to record your daytime activities. Write down what time you exercised. Note the times of day you ate, drank alcohol, and consumed caffeine. Did you have a particularly stressful day? How late did you stay up? What did you do the last few hours before bedtime?

Start to relate your daytime activities to your sleep patterns. You should start to see the correlation between them and be able to identify the lifestyle changes that can help.

Week Three:

Make some adjustments in your daily routine that are conducive to helping you sleep well. Give yourself time to wind down from the stimulating events of the day (it's a bit like cooling down after working out). Three hours before bedtime is a good cut-off point for ingesting heavy meals, doing strenuous workouts, drinking alcohol, and listening to rousing music. Instead, spend your evenings engaging in relaxing activities such as yoga, watching an uplifting or funny movie, writing in your journal, engaging in a hobby, or doing enjoyable chores such as sorting through family photographs or brushing the dog. If you have children, relax with them while playing a quiet game or reading them a story.

Come up with some bedtime rituals that establish boundaries between waking time and sleeping time. For instance, you could take a warm bath scented with calming rosemary, drink some soothing herbal tea such as chamomile or valerian, put on a CD of meditative music, or say an end-of-day prayer or personal affirmation.

mattresses matter

Your mattress is one of the most important pieces of furniture you own, and can largely determine the quality of your sleep. Contrary to conventional wisdom, a good mattress is not necessarily a hard mattress. Nor has there been any medical research to prove the need for expensive orthopedic mattresses. Your mattress should, though, be firm enough to support your spine in its natural curve. In other words, when you're lying down, your spine should be aligned in roughly the same position as when you're in a good standing posture. If that's not the case, you may wake up stiff in the morning because your muscles have to work all night to compensate for the lack of support.

The National Organization for Healthy Backs in England recommends trying this test: Lie on your back and try to slide your hand, palm down, beneath your lower back. If there's a large gap, the mattress is probably too hard. If you have to squeeze your hand in, the mattress is likely too soft. You should be able to just slide your hand snugly between your back and the mattress. This is an inexact science, of course. Comfort, personal preference, and health considerations are largely what determine a perfect mattress for you.

You should replace your mattress about every ten years, sooner if you can feel springs or ridges, or if you and your partner unintentionally roll toward the center. When choosing a new mattress, take off your shoes and lie down on several in the store. Don't be shy about spending time on each one. Try lying in all positions, and have your partner lie next to you. A mattress should be big enough to allow both of you room to move freely and comfortably during the night.

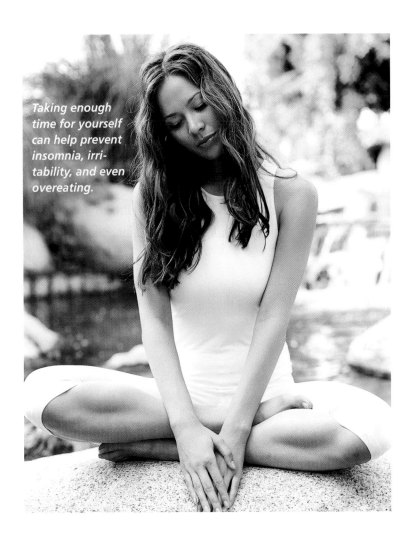

Taking enough time for yourself can help prevent insomnia, irritability, and even overeating.

Week Four:

Give your bedroom a makeover to make it a haven for slumber. Control the brightness with dark shades or curtains. Consider if you need to invest in a new mattress or pillows. Layer your bed with an ample supply of blankets so chilly mornings don't stir you prematurely. Or get a fan to ensure that nights aren't hot and sticky. The gentle whir of a fan can also help block out noises that can keep you awake. For more persistent sounds, consider trying some soft foam earplugs. You could also relocate the television to another room. Unless your job or family circumstances make it imperative that you can be reached during the night, banish the telephone, too.

rest: the pause that refreshes

Sleep is the big "time out," but it's not the only way to regenerate. Paradoxically, while many health experts are urging us to live more mindfully—fully engaged in the moment—society is encouraging us at every turn to multitask. Not too long ago, people would have felt overwhelmed and stressed if they'd been expected to do a number of things at once. Now we feel lazy if we don't. Between our cell phones, pagers, laptops, and personal organizers, we rarely do one task at a time anymore. Heaven forbid that we should consider doing *nothing*. There's some irony in the fact that previous generations fought hard to reduce the work week to 40 hours; now, in our revved-up, fast-tracked world, we're expanding the work week again. We're cramming our lives full of everything except downtime.

Mistake to Avoid: *Although alcohol initially makes you sleepy, you'll eventually experience a rebound arousal effect during the night and wake up after a few hours of sleep. Alcohol also prevents REM (rapid eye movement) sleep, the deepest kind of rest, making whatever sleep you do get less restorative.*

Lacking time to relax and revitalize can eventually lead to a whole host of symptoms. According to Alice Domar, Ph.D., director of the Mind/Body Center for Women's Health at the Harvard Mind/Body Medical Institute and author of *Self-Nurture*, "They might be physical like insomnia or headaches. They might be psychological, like irritability or fatigue. Or they might be behavioral, like emotional outbursts or self-calming behaviors such as smoking or overeating."

Apart from the general pace of 21st-century life, many women spend much of their time caring for others, not to mention juggling family and career. If you don't start taking a little "me" time, you can get to the point where you resent others, and that won't help your relationships, your outlook, or your health. "Getting enough time for themselves is something most women never seem to do," says Domar.

So how much downtime do we need? Your circumstance and temperament will dictate that. Some women need only a few snatched minutes to take a breather and gather their thoughts. Others may need to simplify their entire lives to carve out chunks of time to rest and regenerate.

Make a start by following our four-week plan to learn to take it easier:

Week One:

Every morning when you wake up, take 30 seconds to plan something just for yourself that day, suggests Domar. It might be stopping at a farmer's market and buying a luscious piece of fruit, going for a short walk and literally "smelling the roses," making time to read those e-mail jokes people send you, writing a personal letter, or calling your best friend at the end of the day.

Week Two:

Say no to something every day: the invitation you don't really want to accept, the favor you really don't have time to do, the overtime that's not critical. Use the time you have created in some pleasurable, relaxing way: Read the novel you've been dying to start, plant an herb garden, put on some music, and dance wildly by yourself!

Week Three:

Start taking five-minute mini-relaxation breaks throughout the day at work. Every couple of hours, unplug the phone and sit comfortably. Rest your hand on top of your belly button and feel your abdomen rise and fall an inch as you breathe.

Start making plans for week four when you'll be taking a personal day. Decide on the date, apply for the day off, plan your activities, and arrange a baby-sitter.

Week Four:

Grab an entire day to yourself. Take a drive in the country and stop for lunch in a village café, visit a museum with the awe of a kid, or do a day-long yoga or religious retreat. The important point is to regularly take breaks from your responsibilities, then come back to your life relaxed and refreshed. While you're at it, give some thought to your next vacation and how you'd like to spend it.

get the spa treatment

Had a brutal week? Imagine rewarding yourself with an underwater massage in a private pool filled with flowers. This is just one of the luxuries you can enjoy at a local day spa. These one-stop emporiums of indulgence give you a break from the fast lane to relax and recuperate. In the last ten years, day spas have proliferated—and not just in big cities. You'll find them at free-standing establishments; and also tucked into health clubs, beauty salons, and hotels. The majority have packages including facials, massages, herbal wraps, manicures, and pedicures. And there may be even more exotic offerings, such as Turkish salt scrubs or hot rock rubs. Prices aren't cheap; day packages can range from $200 upward. But the payoff in restorative terms is enormous. Why not ask your family to pool resources and send you to one as a birthday, Mother's Day, or holiday gift?

If you don't have access to, or can't afford, a full-blown spa experience, there may be alternatives in your community. Perhaps there's a natural hot springs where you can soak in therapeutic mineral waters or mud. Bathhouses are a part of many cultures. For example, if there's a large Korean or Japanese community where you live, you may find a no-frills spa where you can soak in the pool and get an excellent massage for a reasonable price.

Don't forget that you can always create the spa experience at home. Stock up on exfoliating scrubs, facial masks, hair conditioners, and luxurious lotions. Perhaps pick a theme for them, such as sea-based or vanilla-scented products. Start with a sparkling clean bathroom supplied with mounds of towels (be lavish—this is a spa!). Create an atmosphere with scented candles and calming music, and turn off the phone. Spend the day in a body-pampering, pleasure-packed, totally relaxing flight of fancy.

vacations

Vacations are another way to recharge. If you think you're too busy for one, think about this: Getting no breaks from telephones and traffic might actually shorten your life. Brooks B. Gump, Ph.D., M.P.H., a psychology professor at the State University of New York, Oswego, found data showing that people who took regular vacations had a 20 percent lower risk of dying from cardiovascular disease in later years. "I suspect vacation benefits come from getting relief from those little daily stressors that constantly raise blood pressure," Gump says.

Time off can be many things to many people. For some it will be a chance to explore cultural activities in a foreign city. Others look for the opportunity to stretch out on a beach with the latest bestseller. An increasing number of women, however, are signing up for action or adventure trips: One statistic states that 63 percent of adventure travelers are women.

Shape® reader Melanie Stern, a health-care professional in Washington, D.C., has been on 17 adventure-travel biking trips over the last 12 years. "When I was in my 20s, I did Club Med," she says. "I outgrew that and wanted a different kind of vacation, something where you're doing a sport and seeing an interesting part of the country."

Women are also white-water rafting in Alaska, snowshoeing in British Columbia, kayaking the coast of Maine, hiking Wyoming's national parks, and rock-climbing in California. These vacations combine drop-dead gorgeous scenery—always a soul refresher—with excitement and the opportunity to challenge oneself. While that may sound contrary to the concept of resting and relaxing, people actually report coming home from these vacations recharged in every way.

But whether your idea of a vacation is a tent in the wilderness or a five-star hotel, it's the break from chronic stress and the chance to have fun with family and friends that does you a world of good.

All of that applies only if you really *do* take a break, though. No fair packing your pager, cell phone, and laptop along with your bathing suit and sunscreen. Vacations are about detaching from work, and when you pack a virtual office, the chances of that happening are remote. Impossible for you to be out of touch for ten days, you say? Ask yourself why. Is your boss really demanding that you stay connected, or are you doing it

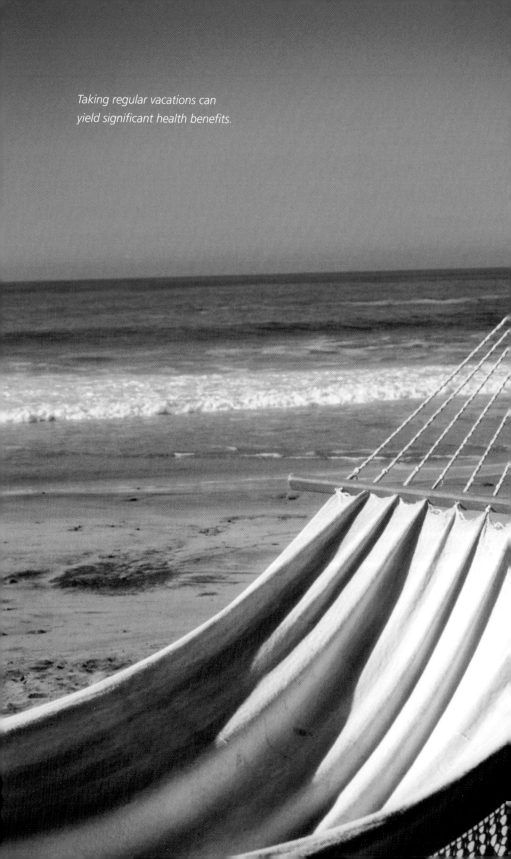

Taking regular vacations can yield significant health benefits.

voluntarily, assuming that your co-workers won't be able to function without you? While it may feel good to be needed, in reality, none of us is as indispensable as we think we are. Remind yourself that all work and no play makes you less productive in the long run, and you'll be doing your colleagues a favor by recharging your batteries.

If your boss demands access to you on your vacation, politely but firmly refuse. Explain that in order to work at your maximum capacity, you need this break. Gump suggests framing it as mental-health time. If you absolutely must stay in touch, do it on your own terms. Agree to call in at prescribed times and no more, and don't give out your number. Who wants to be paged while sipping delicious smoothies on an exotic tropical beach?

It's not just a crisis at the office that can sabotage a vacation. Unexpected weather, travel snafus, and Murphy's Law—which seems to be in effect out of town even more so than at home—can make travel itself so stressful that you may wish you'd never left home. To avoid the counterproductive pitfalls, here are some plan-ahead tips to make the most of your next hard-earned vacation:

Quick Tip: *Vacation turning stressful due to flight delays? Several U.S. airports, including Boston's Logan, Chicago's O'Hare, Las Vegas's McCarran, and Miami International, have on-site health clubs where you can get a day rate to recharge and freshen up. Travelers at Los Angeles International and Dallas/Ft. Worth International can get similar deals at Hilton Hotels, which are just a shuttle bus ride away.*

- *Let the preparation be part of the fun.* Looking through brochures and planning your trip with travel companions can get you in vacation mode before you even leave town.

- *Choose travel companions wisely.* Preexisting friction will worsen away from home.

- *Book big-ticket items such as travel, accommodations, vehicle rentals, and day excursions well in advance* to ensure having choices.

- *Leave everything in order at home and work* so you don't spend your time worrying: there's nothing more tiring.

- *If you're planning an active vacation, start training ahead of time.* Also, break in new shoes you plan to wear.

- *Pack light.* If you can't carry it, it shouldn't go. If you're flying, keep any indispensable items with you in your carry-on bag. Don't let lost luggage ruin your vacation.

- *Once at your destination, be flexible.* Expect some plans to go awry. Getting lost or enduring a spell of bad weather might even lead to memorable experiences.

- *Live by the golden rule when on the road.* An unpleasant exchange with an airline employee can ruin your day. Be agreeable, and you'll get better service and enjoy yourself more.

- *Don't overbook your itinerary,* since everything takes longer in a strange place. Plus, you should definitely allow time for vegging out even on an active vacation. You need your same quota of sleep while you're away.

- *Even on a relaxing vacation, stick to a healthy eating plan* and get some exercise at the hotel gym so you don't go home having gained pounds and inches.

- *Try to get home at least one day before you have to return to the grind.* Unpack slowly, open mail, return calls and e-mails, and ease back into your routine.

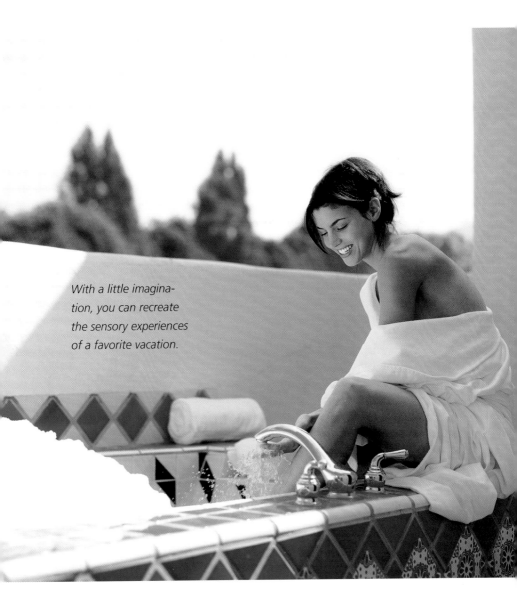

With a little imagina-tion, you can recreate the sensory experiences of a favorite vacation.

- *Incorporate vacation behaviors and activities into your lifestyle.*
  Once home, you may feel depressed because "regular life" seems
  mundane in comparison to your vacation. If you hiked a lot, keep
  doing so at home. If you got more than your usual amount of sleep
  and feel better for it, stick with that habit, too.

jet lag

Anyone who has traveled coast to coast on business or taken an overseas trip knows what havoc crossing time zones can wreak: Sleep eludes you at night, and you feel fatigued and disoriented by day.

Much of the research conducted on the subject of jet lag has been done by sports-medicine organizations, which makes sense. Imagine being an athlete from Florida expected to perform at your peak in the Olympic Games in Sydney; or a World Cup soccer player from France who has to compete in Korea. Sports experts have found that traveling west to east is particularly grueling, since the body's natural cycles are temporarily shortened. The more time zones you cross, the more severe the jet lag; and symptoms of jet lag are most severe two to three days after arrival at the new time zone, after which they diminish gradually.

According to NASA, it takes one day per time zone crossed for your body to recuperate, but there's much you can do help facilitate your body's resynchronization to a new time zone:

- If possible, a week before leaving, start adjusting your sleeping hours by going to bed an hour earlier and getting up an hour later (or vice versa).

- As soon as you get on the plane, set your watch to the time at your destination. Mentally tune in to the new time and act accordingly. In other words, try to sleep on the plane if it's nighttime at your destination.

- Drink lots of water and avoid alcohol and caffeine while traveling.

- Upon arrival, spend as much time outdoors as possible. Natural daylight is the biggest factor in helping reset your body clock.

- Resist napping, and try to stay awake until bedtime in the new time zone.

- Activity and social contact can help accelerate the adjustment.

- Light exercise may help you adjust, but strenuous workouts late in the day can be too stimulating and may keep you awake.

mind tripping

You can't always take off on a vacation whenever you feel the need for a break in your routine, so why not escape for a while to the last great vacation you took? Rachel Harris, Ph.D., a psychologist practicing in New Jersey, and author of *20-Minute Retreats,* recommends a "Vacation Visualization." This is a meditative excursion that can help you recapture the feelings of rest and revitalization you experienced on your last trip. And if there isn't an actual place you want to revisit, use your imagination to create your ideal vacation location.

20-minute vacation visualization

Step 1: Prepare for your journey by getting comfortable and observing your breath for a couple of minutes.

Step 2: Spend the next 15 minutes "on vacation." Let your mind conjure up your favorite spot. "The important thing is to remember as many sensory details as you can," says Harris. Experience the warmth of the sun or the sting of crisp mountain air on your cheeks, scrunch the sand between your toes, or feel the cobblestone street under your shoes. Are there exotic animal, bird, and insect noises? Do the people who inhabit your vacation world speak with a different accent or in a foreign language? What about the structures and the way the light plays upon

Quick Tip: *Doing aerobic activities between 4 and 6 P.M. might help you sleep. Aerobic workouts raise your body temperature and metabolism; sleep occurs with the opposite. When you exercise in the late afternoon/early evening, you experience a steep drop in temperature by the time you go to sleep, potentially making your snooze time deeper and more satisfying.*

them? "Smell is particularly evocative," says Harris. Do you recall the fragrance of the night-scented blossoms outside your window, the tang of salty air, or the aroma of the baking bread from the little café in the square? The key is to immerse yourself in as much detail as possible. "You're doing more than just remembering a relaxing vacation moment," says Harris. "With all the sensory richness, you're actually creating the experience in the present."

Step 3: Finally, spend about three minutes on the return journey. Reenter the here-and-now, bringing with you feelings of peace, relaxation, and rejuvenation.

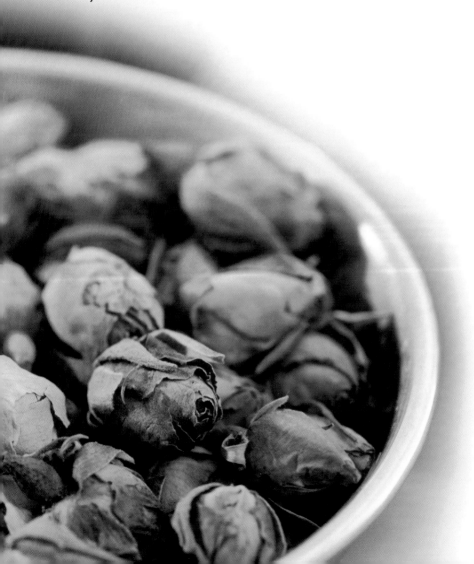

rest and exercise: recover and rebuild

You need to factor in rest even when it comes to exercising. Muscles require time to recover between workouts, so in addition to getting enough daily sleep, you also need to build recovery time into your regimen so that you can make strength gains. When you first begin working out, you'll be using lighter weights, so you won't need as much recovery time between workout sessions—a day may be sufficient. And you may be able to handle three total body strength-training days weekly in addition to your regular cardio activity.

As you progress to heavier weights and more challenging workouts, however, you'll need more recovery time—decreasing weight training to two days per week because you may need 48 hours to recover. In addition, lifting heavier weights will require that you lengthen rest time between multiple sets of exercise: Instead of resting 45 seconds to one minute between sets, you may need up to two minutes between them, plus more rest between exercises. As your intensity increases, you'll need to build in even more rest days.

The same goes for cardio training. For example, if you're currently doing five cardio sessions per week, you may need to decrease it to four and take a day off after a very strenuous workout.

It may seem paradoxical that fewer workouts and longer rest periods can produce more progress, but it's true. If you fail to allow your muscles and body systems time to recover during and after tough workouts, chances are you'll stay fatigued and overtrained . . . and be disappointed with your results.

> **Mistake to Avoid:**
>
> *Don't pass on a vacation citing lack of money or time. Even a three-day camping trip at a local state park can yield restorative results.*

the recess workout

Sometimes just changing your routine can prevent you from getting tired of your workout regimen. Playing, just like you did as a kid, can energize you. Get strong and loose, but most of all, have fun with this playground-inspired workout. Do it with other kidlike adults for an extra jolt of fun—after all, recess wouldn't be recess if it didn't involve playing with others.

This workout is meant to complement a traditional cardiovascular and strength-training program. So you can do these exercises twice a week on nonconsecutive days if you're not in training, but if you're actively involved in a sport or are currently training, one day a week is enough. Don't do them at the expense of your rest days.

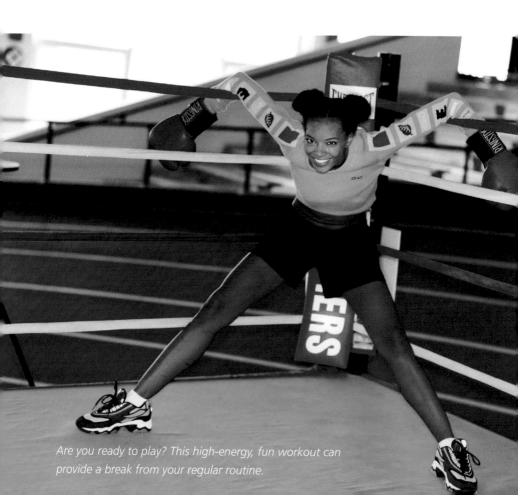

Are you ready to play? This high-energy, fun workout can provide a break from your regular routine.

the plan

Begin with the recommended number of reps and sets listed in each caption, and then feel free to add sets as you become more familiar with the program. If you're just starting out with this kind of training, take breaks in between the exercises as you need to.

Begin with five minutes of low-intensity exercises, such as walking briskly, climbing a flight of stairs, or using a stair stepper or another piece of home cardio equipment. To cool down, stretch all major muscles, especially the calves. Hold each stretch to the point of mild tension for 20–30 seconds, but don't bounce.

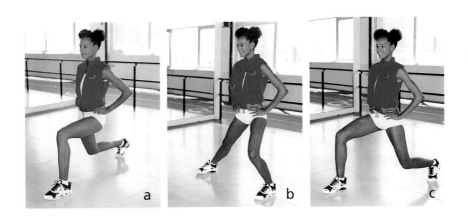

1. Spokes of a Wheel. *Stand with feet hip-width apart, legs straight (not locked), hands on hips. Lunge forward with your left leg, bending your knees. Left knee should be above left ankle, not past toes; right knee should come close to the floor, heel lifted (a). Push back to starting position, keeping torso straight. Repeat with right leg. Continue alternating in these directions: 45 degrees forward (on a diagonal, keeping supporting leg straight), directly sideways (b), 45 degrees backward (diagonal) (c), directly backward. Do 3–5 sets (one set equals all 5 lunges with both feet).*

Improves agility and coordination in all directions; strengthens legs and butt.

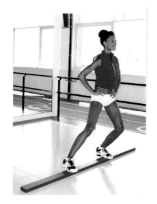

2. Defensive Slides. Balance on a 2" by 4" by 5' beam of wood, feet shoulder-width apart, knees bent in a quarter-squat position, balancing on the balls of your feet. Slide quickly to the left, moving feet in the same direction, keeping them shoulder-width apart. Remain in the squat position as you slide. Then change direction, going to the right. Slide 2–4 times in each direction. To progress: Do 10–15 reps of thigh parallel squats before you slide; you may also add momentum, sliding faster and allowing some space under the balls of your feet while you move.

Develops balance; builds speed and agility; works hips and legs.

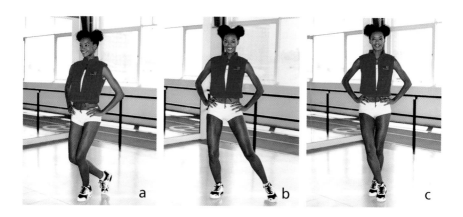

a   b   c

3. Carioca. Start with feet slightly apart, legs straight (not locked), hands on hips. Cross left foot in front of right (a); step out sideways with right foot so legs are hip-width apart, shifting weight toward the right (b). Cross left foot behind right (c) and step out sideways with right foot again (b). Continue this grapevine pattern, staying light on the balls of your feet. Hips should follow feet. Focus on taking quick, small steps. Repeat 4–6 times in each direction. To progress: Do this on a beam to improve balance.

Improves agility, coordination, and speed.

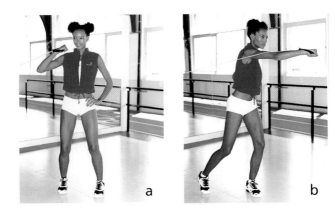

a   b

4. Rotary Push. *Put a resistance tube through a doorjamb at waist height and shut the door. Stand with your right side to the door, facing 45 degrees to the left. Keep feet about hip-width apart. Hold the tube handle in your right hand as if you're going to throw a shot put, that is, close to your right shoulder, palm facing in and elbow bent so you have tension on the tube (a). Pivot your legs and hips away from the door; then let your entire body rotate to the left as you punch out and up, straightening your right arm (b). Bend right elbow and return to starting position. Do one set of 10–15 reps; then switch to left side. Do two sets on each side.*

    Improves punching and pushing power; strengthens chest, shoulders, and arms.

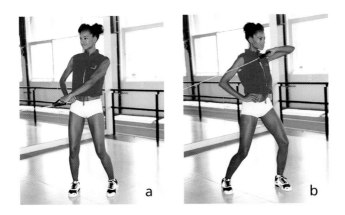

a   b

5. Rotary Pull. *Put a resistance tube through a doorjamb at waist height and shut the door. Stand with your right side to the door, facing 45 degrees to the left. Keep feet about hip-width apart. Hold the tube handle in your left hand, arm straight but not locked, palm down. Rotate body toward the door (a).*

Pushing off the left foot and keeping knees flexed, bend your left elbow toward your left shoulder as if drawing back an arrow from a bow. Your body will rotate away from the door as you pull (b). Use your hips and torso to create the rotation; your arm will follow. Slowly release the tube and return to starting position. Do 10–15 reps; then switch sides. Do two sets on each side. *Improves pulling power; strengthens back, shoulders, and arms.*

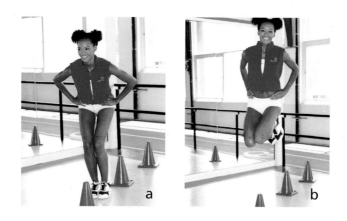

6. Cone Jumps. Set up 3–4 cones (or 3–4 filled one-gallon bottles of water) in a row with 3–4 feet between them. Bend both knees, keeping your feet together, and crouch (a). Then do a double-leg jump over each cone (b). Try to jump as quickly and as high as you can, but land softly. When you get to the end of the row, turn around and jump back to the first cone. Begin with 1–2 sets and work up to 4 sets of 10 jumps, resting 30–60 seconds between sets. *Develops power in the buttocks, quadriceps, and calves.*

the program in action

The horse ran away with her once, she was scared on several occasions, and she thought about quitting at least ten times the first day alone. For Jane Wolfberg, this vacation was nothing like her quiet life as a legal secretary in Los Angeles. Wolfberg had signed up to learn how to ride in Scotland because she'd always loved horses. As a child, she'd never had the opportunity to take more than an occasional pony ride. But now as a professional with the financial wherewithal, she couldn't think of a reason not to learn to ride better. So she researched to find the most challenging trip that seemed to suit her skill level. "I didn't just want to be on a trail ride," she says. "I wanted a challenge I can't normally get in life."

Wolfberg made it through that first day, and the second. And then it happened. She gave the command and the horse cantered on cue. It felt like lifting off. Then there were the drumming hooves underneath her. More than that, it was if Scotland itself opened up—in the land she saw shades of green previously unknown to her, and marveled at the beauty of the heather's pinkish-purple blooms. The stinging sea breeze took her breath away; the grime of leather oil and dirt got under her fingernails. The shared thrill brought her close to her fellow riders on the trip. They all rode until the sun finally set (at this far northern latitude) at 11 P.M.

"I felt really alive. I realized then there's a part of me that had been craving this," says Wolfberg whose fifth international riding trip was to Italy. "On these trips, all my senses are completely in the moment. There are very few things I do in the rest of my life that are like that."

But she wants them to be. Her first step since her epiphany in Scotland was to join a riding club at home, and now she rides regularly.

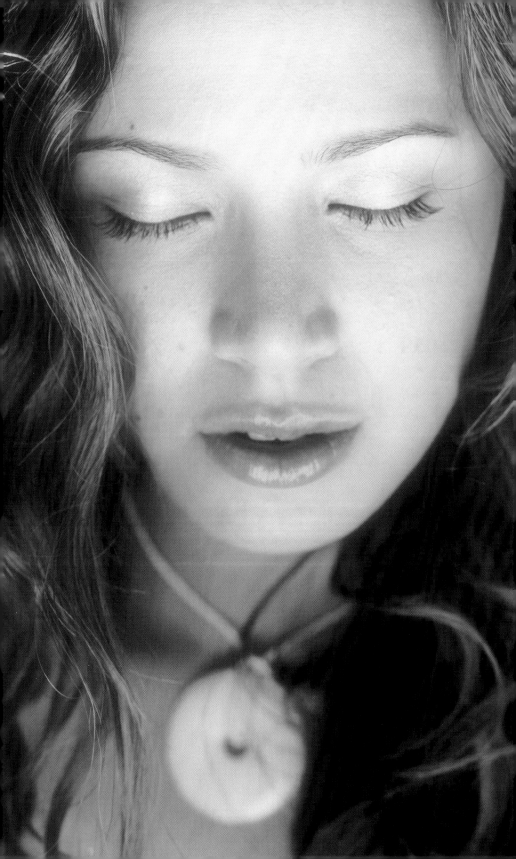

chapter five
your emotions

Mistake to Avoid: *Don't postpone
happiness until you acquire one more
thing—such as career success, a mate,
a family, or financial security. Your desire
to succeed may keep you rushing from
one achievement to the next with no
end in sight . . . and happiness may
elude you forever.*

what you'll learn

Shape's approach to your emotions is that we want to do much better than just survive—we want to find joy—and that a healthy, optimistic mind-set and rich relationships are key elements in achieving a healthy body. Using this chapter you'll learn techniques to:

- be happy by cultivating optimism
- soothe stress
- slow down to get more out of every day
- build intimate connections with key people
- ignite passions
- confront fears and phobias
- kick bad habits that sap emotional health

Quick Tip: *Smile!*
Before you laugh off that advice as a greeting-card platitude, consider the research. Data from Oxford University in England suggests that smiling promotes trust among strangers and boosts levels of cooperation—results that can de-stress your day. Plus, a long-term study conducted by researchers at University of California at Berkeley revealed that women who smiled broadly in their college yearbook pictures taken 30 years ago went on to have the most successful relationships and careers.

how you'll do it

When the Founding Fathers promised us the pursuit of happiness, they must have known that the hard part was actually catching up with it. For a long time, psychologists weren't much help in this pursuit, focusing instead on the things that made us unhappy. In fact, throughout much of the 20th century, mental-health professionals agreed with Sigmund Freud that optimism was an illusion that kept the masses happy, and only those who were coldly realistic were psychologically balanced. Psychologists and therapists concentrated on dysfunction, researching and treating everything from depression to panic disorders while paying little attention to the mentally healthy and the content—and what made them that way.

Today, there's a relatively new field called Positive Psychology that has a more rose-colored focus: Practitioners believe that learning how to promote joy and happiness will, in turn, lessen negative feelings and depression. They also believe that negative thinking is itself the disease—rather than just a symptom of depression. Simply put, Positive Psychology attempts to discover what works and how to develop it, rather than concentrate on what isn't working.

create the life you want by writing your personal story

Elaine M. Sullivan, M.Ed., LPC, LMFT, is a psychotherapist who conducts personal and professional growth and wellness workshops, nationally and internationally. Here is one of her journaling exercises:

1. *Divide your life into decades, allowing one full page for each.* Briefly describe the highs and the lows that marked that time in your life. Think about these pivotal times, and write down something you learned about yourself during each one and a quality you gained as a result.

2. *Write down how you felt about yourself during each decade:* physically (body confidence/image), socially (relationships), occupationally, emotionally, intellectually, and spiritually.

3. *Record one memory you associate with each of these words:* laughter, sadness, anger, fear, joy, grief, and kindness.

4. *Imagine all the fresh, white pages ahead in Volume II of your life story,* and describe yourself—as the best you can be—five years from today. Where would you like to see yourself physically, socially, professionally, emotionally, intellectually, and spiritually?

5. *Write down what you envision to be the potential "highs" in your life.* Think about all the different areas in your life where you've enjoyed success.

6. *Let go of old labels* ("I'm overweight, untalented, stuck in my job") and envision yourself as you'd like to be ("I'm healthy, creative, in a job I enjoy"). Brainstorm concrete ways to make these things happen (for example, see a nutritionist, start walking, take an art class, or research interesting jobs) and write them down. This is how to begin creating Volume II, the life you want to be living.

quiz: is stress putting your health at risk?

Everyone reacts to stress differently. What overwhelms one person may be a motivating challenge to another. It's not the situation that can affect your health; it's how you perceive it. To see if your reactions can compromise your health, take our quiz.

YES NO

___ ___ 1. I get lots of tension headaches.

___ ___ 2. I often breathe faster and my heart "races."

___ ___ 3. I clench my jaw or grind my teeth.

___ ___ 4. I routinely "feel" stressed.

___ ___ 5. I tend to suffer from gastrointestinal symptoms such as diarrhea.

___ ___ 6. I often experience muscle tension, such as hunched shoulders or a stiff neck.

___ ___ 7. I often feel nervous or jittery.

___ ___ 8. I perspire a lot, or get chills and clammy hands.

___ ___ 9. I easily become upset, angry, irritable, or impatient.

SCORING

Some of these answers could indicate other medical problems, but if you answered yes to more than three of them, it may mean that you react to stress in harmful ways. You need to learn coping skills and long-term relaxation techniques. For immediate stress relief, sit quietly, taking slow, deep breaths. Relax your shoulders and jaw; visualize a peaceful place, or listen to calming music. Concentrate on changing your mind-set, too: If you're bugged by a crying baby at the next table, consider how hard it is for infants to communicate their needs; if you're worried about an upcoming exam, remind yourself that you almost always do fine.

"In the past, we were too preoccupied with repairing damage, when our focus should be on building strength and resilience," says Positive Psychology advocate Martin Seligman, Ph.D., professor of psychology at the University of Pennsylvania and former president of the American Psychological Association.

In recent years, researchers have developed what amounts to a science of happiness, and now they, too, are giving chase to it. It turns out that happiness is not all that elusive. In a survey of almost 2,500 men and women conducted by the National Opinion Research Center, three out of ten Americans say they're "very happy," and another six say they're "pretty happy." Truly pity the lone soul who claims to be "not too happy."

The causes of all this contentment may surprise you. Another survey conducted by the University of Missouri reports that popularity, influence, luxury, and money—traditional elements of the "American Dream"—appear at the very bottom of the lists of what makes us happy. The common wisdom that wealth doesn't buy happiness is, apparently, right on the money.

The study's findings on those things that *do* make us happy largely concur with what David Myers, Ph.D., psychology professor at Michigan's Hope College and author of *The Pursuit of Happiness* has discovered in his own research. He found that happy people share four main characteristics: They have high self-esteem, they feel in control, they're sociable and extroverted, and they're optimistic. The Missouri survey adds feeling competent to that list. And there's more: Myers has also found that we can make ourselves happy by acting as if we already are. "Going through the motions," he says, "can generate the emotions."

In fact, you can actually improve your mood by cultivating optimism—essentially the inclination to put a positive spin on life's actions and events. Although there is debate about whether optimism and pessimism are inherited traits (some experts say that your outlook is 25 to 50 percent genetic), the argument is largely moot. Experts do agree that even the most die-hard pessimists have the ability to become more optimistic and improve their emotional health while they're at it.

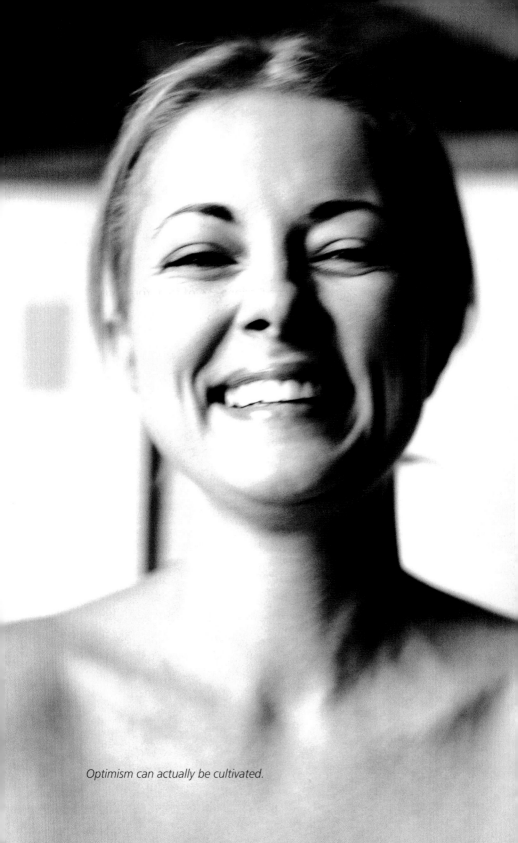

Optimism can actually be cultivated.

To do this, you need to know how optimists act. Let's be clear: A person who thinks every lottery ticket is the big winner isn't optimistic—she's naive! Three characteristics define a true optimist, according to Peg Baim, M.S., N.P., an associate in medicine at Harvard Medical School who teaches physicians how to help patients via optimism. The traits are:

1. She is a problem solver who takes charge of her life. If she hates her job, she won't just spend the next few years complaining about it. She'll research other careers, network with friends, and take classes that might lead to more appealing work.

    Shape® reader Kathleen Piccione, 32, of New York could be the "problem-solver" poster girl. Some years ago, she took what seemed to be a perfect position in suburban New Jersey. "But it turned out to be a horrible dead-end job," she says. "I focused on what I really wanted and discovered it was the excitement of working both in finance and in nearby New York City." After lots of job hunting (and no settling), she found a great job in a top investment-banking firm "in the city I love."

2. When something happens that she can't control, she examines the situation to find meaning. If her boyfriend dumps her, she'll acknowledge through her tears that although the relationship wasn't meant to be, it was a valuable life experience. If she loses a family member, she'll emerge from her grief with a new appreciation of how precious life is.

3. She doesn't distort problems. She doesn't blame herself, nor does she think her problems are chronic or unsolvable (the way a classic pessimist does). She tends to see a situation for what it is. Instead of viewing her tough new boss as impossible, she'll appreciate being challenged and having the opportunity to learn and grow.

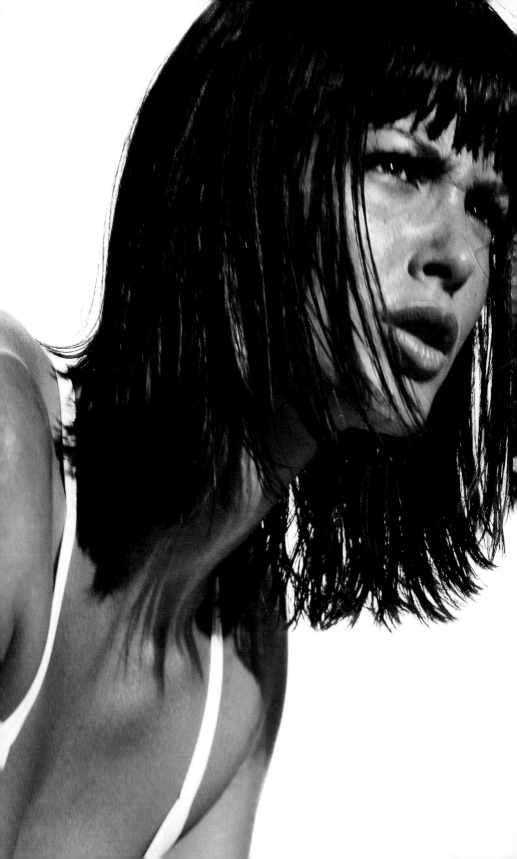

a healthy mind
means a healthy body

It's not just your emotional well-being that benefits when you're optimistic. Findings show that focusing on the upside will also make you healthier and help you live longer. A study tracking more than 800 patients from the Mayo Clinic found that the pessimists (determined by personality testing) had a 19 percent higher mortality rate than optimists. Another study conducted by Wilkes University and a Veterans Administration medical center in New Jersey showed that those who were classified as pessimists had lower levels of an antibody that fights colds and other illnesses.

Nevertheless, psychologists make the point that while optimism is important to your health, it is by no means the only factor involved. If you have strep throat, antibiotics are going to improve your health more than optimism will. So a smart-thinking optimist would seek medical assistance to treat the strep throat—and then have faith that the next time she's exposed to a contagious bug, her optimism-enhanced immune system will help fight it off.

Further, adds Baim, because optimists are excellent problems solvers, they're more likely to seek solutions that lead to good health. "If you get a heart attack, you're probably more likely to exercise afterward," she says.

What if you really do have a crisis? Putting it into a favorable light can seem like denial. And isn't denial bad for the psyche? Not necessarily, says the research. A review article by University of California at Los Angeles (UCLA) psychologist Shelley Taylor, Ph.D., who has spent more than 20 years studying optimism and pessimism in breast-cancer and AIDS patients, found that even unrealistic optimism (like believing your cancer will go into remission even when there's little chance of it) is linked to better health.

the stress factor

The reason why optimists are physically healthier than pessimists might be explained by the fact that optimists "experience less stress, and therefore suffer less from stress physiology," says Harvard's Baim.

You're familiar with stress, aren't you? The deadline you can't possibly meet, the never-satisfied boss, the "you-don't-deserve-him" mother-in-law: We all know how pressure and aggravation can make us feel—not only emotionally, but physically—the racing heartbeat, the churning gut, the sweaty palms, the dry mouth. Mental stress has always had its physical component. In fact, that's what the stress response is: the visceral priming of the body to either fight or flee from a perceived danger. But even low-level stress, the kind that's so constant you consider it normal, can cause aches and pains that you might not attribute to emotions.

"Many people who have stress-related pain aren't even aware of what they're fearful or angry about," says Ian Wickramasekera, Ph.D., clinical professor of psychiatry at Stanford University Medical School. By some estimates, half of the patients whom doctors see for various common body aches are actually expressing psychological distress through physical pain. Stress experts across the country saw evidence of this after the terrorist attacks on September 11, 2001.

"In 30 years of specializing in stress-related diseases, I've never seen more flare-ups of physical pain, even in people who'd been free of symptoms for years," says Wickramasekera.

The source of stress-related pain lies in the brain, which, when you feel under the gun, triggers the release of cortisol, adrenaline, and other hormones that prepare the body for action by, for example, increasing heart rate, blood pressure, and respiration. Less noticeably, these hormones also make muscles tense up, which can cause aches and irritate nerves. The lower back, neck, shoulders, head, and jaw are particularly prone to stress-related pain.

Chronic stress can also impair long-term health. Stress hormones work on the part of the brain responsible for memory formation. While these hormones help sharpen memory in the short term, long-term, repeated exposures can lead to memory loss. And increased cortisol turns on fat-cell storage throughout the body, especially in the abdomen.

> **Mistake to Avoid:**
>
> *Don't be too serious. It's impossible to feel stressed or anxious when you're doubled over in a fit of giggles. Plus, laughter is good medicine. Studies have shown that laughter not only relieves tension, but actually improves immune functions and helps us cope with pain.*

Studies have shown that women feel stress more often than men. According to the American Psychological Association, women tend to repetitively and passively dwell on symptoms, causes, and consequences of distress, which leads to longer and more severe bouts of stress. Also, women tend to worry in a more global way. Whereas a man might fret about something actual and specific—such as the fact that he's just been passed over for a promotion—a woman will tend to worry abstractly about her job, her weight, plus the well-being of every member of her extended family.

More specifically, women apparently are concerned about their daughters. A 2001 study at the University of Michigan Institute for Social Research found that nearly two-thirds of midlife women thought that their adult daughters were more successful in their careers, yet they were less happy than their mothers had been at the same age. Many of the mothers felt that the strains of combining work and family, the stress of professional careers, and the difficulties accompanying nontraditional families—including stepfamilies and single motherhood—were problems unique to our modern society.

slow down

Being harried is a surefire recipe for stress. Yet becoming deliberate and unhurried is not easy to do. "The main cause of stress is an overactive mind," says Joseph Bailey, M.A., a psychologist in St. Paul, Minnesota, and author of *The Speed Trap: How to Avoid the Frenzy of the Fast Lane.* "People who are juggling all their to-do lists in their minds, who are worrying about the future or thinking about the past, are caught up in a vicious cycle of thoughts that create stress. When we slow down on the inside, we immediately reduce our stress."

We can help calm our racing minds by employing calming techniques and generally taking care of ourselves. Yet when we've become accustomed to running at breakneck speed, we often put self-care at the bottom of our to-do lists. Then, when we're overly busy, "we slip back into our old addictive habits," Bailey says. We overeat, we skip workouts and meditation sessions, and we may even turn to cigarettes, alcohol, or drugs for respite." To be healthy, we need to make time for what's truly important. Sometimes, of course, making time for what's of value to you requires that you first figure out *what's* important to you. Too many of us put our jobs first and squeeze everything else into the scant time left over. But that's not the best way to prioritize, says Stephanie Winston, author of *Getting Out from Under: Redefining Your Priorities in an Overwhelming World*. Winston recommends writing a list of your top five priorities and comparing them with your current day-to-day life. "If you find that your real life and your desired life are just too far apart, sit down and give some thought to how you can redirect that balance so your real life reflects more of the things you hope for."

It's also important to figure out what causes the most stress in your life: Is it your three-hour-a-day commute? Your son's four-times-a-week soccer games? The evening MBA program you're trying to complete in two years? Probably, only one or two things are really overwhelming you. And, experts say, the clearer you can be about what's causing you stress, the easier it will be to create a strategy for dealing with it.

After you've gotten a firm handle on your priorities and your stressors, you may find that slowing down will require a major change—perhaps a new job to lessen your commute. Reducing stress could also require you to learn to say no more often, let the phone ring and return calls at your convenience, and read your e-mail only twice a day. When you do begin to slow down, life-changing decisions will be less daunting. Bailey says, "When you calm down on the inside, then you begin to access wisdom and common sense, and you begin to see how to make changes in your lifestyle that would complement a healthy life."

Almost all of the subject matter that this book covers can help you live a more manageable life with less stress: exercising regularly, eating a healthy diet, getting sufficient sleep, nurturing your spirituality, feeling good about your body, and having a satisfying career. In addition, here is a four-week plan with specific techniques you can use to become calm, relaxed, and focused in the moment:

Week One:

Find yourself a stress talisman to keep in your pocket. This will serve as a physical reminder of your desire to be calm. When you feel stress bubbling up, touch the object. It can be a smooth pebble you find on a walk or something special that you buy. Many cultures have long traditions of employing such objects. The Greeks use worry beads and, in slang, sometimes refer to them as "cigarettes," since they provide a calming alternative when someone is trying to quit smoking. And the Chinese have small metal balls—often called stress balls or worry balls—that you can roll

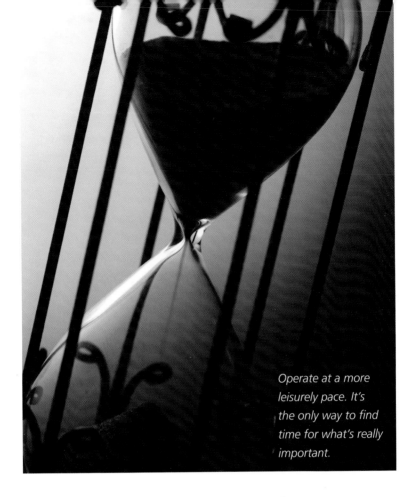

Operate at a more leisurely pace. It's the only way to find time for what's really important.

around in your hand. You'll find them in Asian import stores. Your talisman could also be worn on a chain around your neck, as could anything that you designate as your personal de-stressing trigger.

Week Two:

Equip yourself for waiting. You know the deal—you rush to keep your appointment, and then you sit in the doctor's reception area for 45 minutes with nothing to occupy you but some old *National Geographic*s and your growing impatience. We live in a "hurry up and wait" society, so why not accept the inevitable? Try these tips to prepare yourself so you can use downtime to de-stress:

- *Pack a book.* Make it escapist fare: a mystery or a romance novel.

- *Knit or crochet.* These crafting activities can be immensely satisfying and relaxing. Plus, you'll have handmade gifts to show for your waiting time!

- *Write.* Use the time for journaling, or drop a note to a friend you haven't seen in a while.

- *Listen up.* Get a personal CD player and listen to your choice of soothing or uplifting music. Or, listen to books on tape.

- *Meditate.* You can do this anywhere: Just sit comfortably, close your eyes, focus on your breathing, and let go of your thoughts. If it helps, silently repeat a word or phrase.

Week Three:

Learn to relax the muscles in your neck and face. We carry a lot of tension in these areas when we're stressed. These are short, do-anywhere techniques.

Give your neck muscles an all-around stretch one step at a time. While sitting erect, lower your chin to your chest, letting the weight of your head gently stretch tense muscles at the back of the neck. Hold for 15 seconds. Next, gently let your head drop toward one shoulder. Hold for 15 seconds and repeat on the other side.

Do a self-massage of the muscles in your face and neck. Start by gently pressing your fingers on both sides of your face around the hinge of your jaw, rubbing the area in a circular motion, then kneading the skin with your fingers. Next, move your hands to the area just behind the jaw and below the ears, massaging gently as you slowly slide your hands down your back to the base of your shoulders.

Open your jaw as wide as you can, hold for a few moments, then gradually let it relax.

Week Four:

Take a one-hour stress break. An hour is a lot of time in a fast-paced world. This week, carve out a full 60 minutes from your schedule to spend entirely on nurturing yourself. You may find it difficult at first to indulge in this much time in one block. Focus on how you want to spend that guilt-free hour—it could be anything from giving yourself a pedicure, to taking a walk, to listening to your favorite music. Arrange your time so you won't be interrupted, and be mentally and emotionally present in your chosen activity.

cry, baby

"Laugh, and the world laughs with you; cry, and you cry alone." The old saying is clever but incomplete. When we cry, others can't help but respond in some way, because tears are a means of expressing what we can't say with words. Tears often represent pain, fear, joy, or grief. Most often they're a plea for help.

According to the *British Journal of Social Psychology*, when we cry, we admit to being overwhelmed and implicitly appeal to others to help us reclaim our power, thus creating a shared goal. In contrast, some clinically depressed people never cry. Like a severely neglected infant who no longer believes it will be picked up, they don't see the point.

Crying can be a healthy, social impulse, and almost everyone agrees that it can make us feel better. Still, it's not always appropriate—for example, crying in the workplace can lead to discomfort or embarrassment for everyone involved and can make you look powerless or manipulative.

Crying has other purposes, of course. Our ancestors used it for everything from pagan rituals to aesthetic experiences. Now we see a good cry as a health measure: a "cooling system" for overheated nerves, a release. Our society also tends to romanticize tears as an expression of deep emotion—sensual and erotically powerful. Most often, though, we cry to convey our needs.

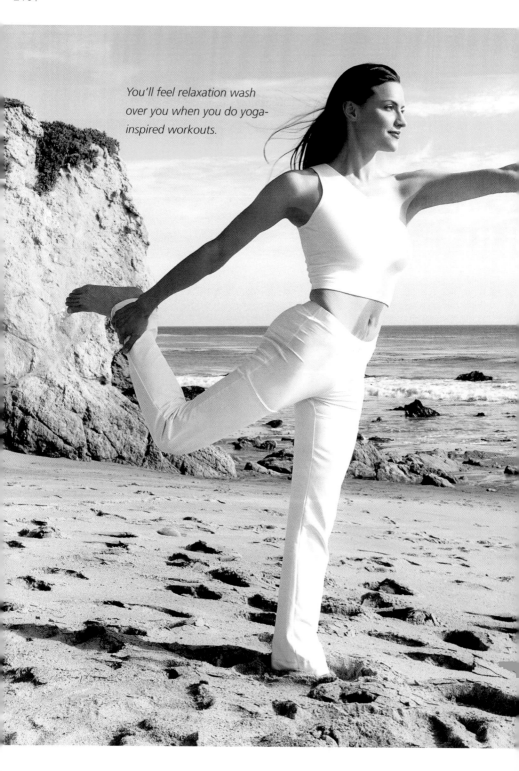

You'll feel relaxation wash over you when you do yoga-inspired workouts.

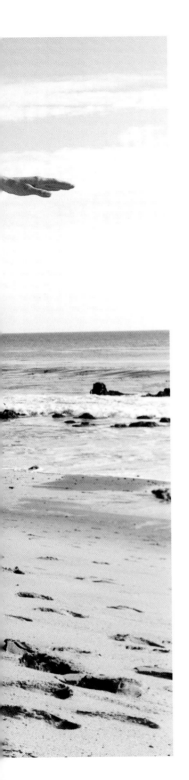

the lean and serene workout

As we've said many times, exercise can help keep your emotions in equilibrium. There's little else that has such an immediate effect in terms of boosting your moods. But exercise doesn't have to be fast, furious, and loud to relieve stress and make you feel good. There's another route you can take: a kinder, gentler approach that's all the rage in Hollywood. By fusing yoga, Pilates, and ballet, fitness authority Karen Voight has designed a workout that not only results in wonderful body changes, but is also a great stress-melter. "You'll gain focus, clarity, and perspective," Voight says. Doing this workout amid the tranquility of nature is another way to make it even more potent.

the plan

Do this workout 3 times a week. Perform 4–6 reps of each move in the order shown. Get into and out of position at a steady pace, and use proper form. It should take 20 minutes to do all 6 moves. When you can comfortably do 6 reps, progress to 8 reps.

Warm up with 10 minutes of walking, stair climbing, or other low-intensity activity. Cool down by stretching all major muscles, holding each stretch to the point of mild tension for 30 seconds, without bouncing.

Supplement this workout with 30–45 minutes of aerobic activity 3–5 times a week.

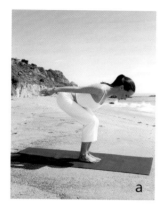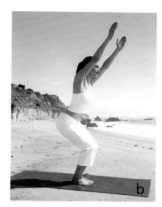

1. Floating Chair. *Standing with your feet, knees, and ankles together, shift your body weight toward your heels, bend your knees, and hinge forward at the hips until your chest nearly touches your thighs. Extend your arms behind you in line with your torso, palms facing in (a). Squeeze your shoulder blades together, then slowly rotate your arms out, turn your palms in, and bring your arms straight up as you lift your torso up to a 45-degree angle, maintaining the chair position (b). Return to starting position and repeat.*

Strengthens quadriceps, abdominals, lower- and upper-back muscles, and shoulders.

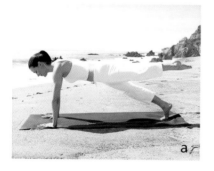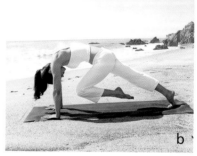

2. Knee-to-Chest Plank. *Start on hands and knees, wrists in line with shoulders, abs tight, hips squared. Extend legs straight back, balancing on balls of feet, ankles together (beginners can stay on knees). Lift left leg to hip height (a). Pull left knee toward chest; use abs to round spine, bringing nose toward left knee (b). Straighten leg and spine, repeat for reps; switch legs.*

Strengthens abdominals, back, buttocks, shoulders, and arms; stretches back and buttocks.

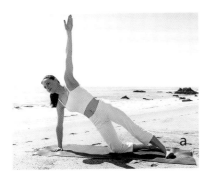 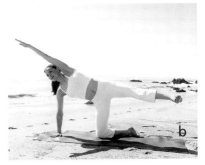

3. Side Reach and Lift. With right hand on ground directly under shoulder, arm straight, and shoulders back, kneel on right knee with right foot behind. Extend left leg, left foot flexed, inner part on the ground. Contract abs and extend left arm up (a). Push into ground with right hand as you lift left leg to hip height and lower left arm toward head (b). Return to starting position. Do reps; switch sides.

　　Strengthens arms, abdominals, back, hip abductors, thighs, and buttocks.

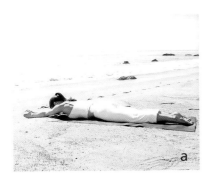 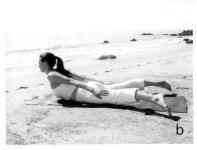

4. Moving Locust. Lie facedown on ground, knees and ankles together, and palms touching above head, arms straight. Contract abdominals so front of hipbones are against ground and navel is off ground (a). Squeeze shoulder blades down to lift head, chest, and shoulders, then sweep arms out and around onto back of thighs. Meanwhile, use buttock muscles to lift legs off ground, palms and feet together; repeat.

　　Strengthens back and abdominal muscles, buttocks, hip abductors, hip adductors, and shoulders; stretches chest and front shoulders.

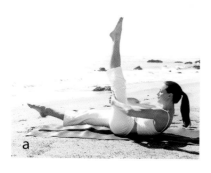 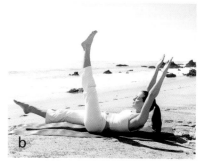

5. Scissor Switch. *Lying faceup on ground, lift left leg up to 90 degrees and extend right leg, slightly lifted off ground. Put hands behind left thigh. Inhale; lift head, neck, and shoulder blades off ground. Exhale, using abs and arms to lift chest toward left knee by bending elbows (a). Hold torso and leg positions as you float arms up and behind head (b). Inhale, switching legs as you bring hands behind right thigh. Continue to float arms behind head and alternate legs, exhaling and lifting chest toward knee, for all reps.*

Strengthens abdominals, biceps, and thighs.

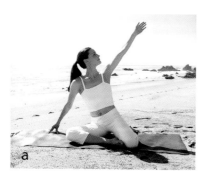 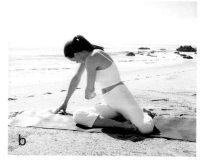

6. Spiraling Ab Twist. *Sit on right hip, knees bent, right ankle lining up with groin, left ankle behind you. Put right fingertips on ground in line with right shoulder; extend left arm up at a diagonal (a). Inhale as you press left arm back to feel a torso stretch. Exhale as you contract abs. Curl shoulders inward, rotating to the right, moving left forearm between right hand and hip (b). Inhale, and return to starting position. Do reps; switch sides.*

Strengthens abdominals, particularly obliques; stretches front of hips and quadriceps, shoulders, and middle back.

get intimate

When you de-stress and make time for yourself, you'll also improve your relationships with your friends, mate, and family. "When our minds slow down, we're more present, we're better listeners, we talk from the heart, and we experience more intimacy," says Joseph Bailey, M.A. Impatience is a by-product of a hurried life, and it can really inflict damage on relationships. When you're rushed and impatient, you become irritated and judgmental, and that creates distance between you and other people.

Not only does being less stressed help our relationships, but close ties help us tolerate stress better. In Chapter 3, "Your Spirituality," we discuss how connectedness helps nurture our souls, but intimate friendships can also soothe our minds.

"Friends are great at reducing each other's frustration and anxiety," says Sandy Sheehy, author of *Connecting: The Enduring Power of Female Friendship*. "Because she respects and admires you, she reflects back an image of a strong, healthy woman. Her respect and admiration encourage you to stick with the habits that will keep you strong and healthy."

Quick Tip: *Get help when you need it. If you can't shake pessimism or negative thinking, seek professional help. Consider cognitive therapy, which focuses on changing your unfavorable thoughts and beliefs into positive ones, which in turn improves your mood.*

Talking to your friend about the source of your stress—for example, when your boyfriend takes you for granted—and her acknowledgment of it, is often enough to make you feel better. Intimate conversation is the essence of female friendship, while the opposite is true of most male friendships. Men tend to do things together. Women delve into relationships by talking, telling secrets, and revealing profoundly personal things, whereas male buddies are generally busy with a mutual activity, and talk is likely to be about something impersonal, such as sports or work.

So recognize the importance of your friendships. College age to 40 is prime time for making friends, says Sheehy. But it's also when women undergo job changes, marriage, and motherhood—transitions that make holding on to friendships a challenge. To ensure that a new friend will become a beloved old one, find a way to nurture the friendship—even if it's only with e-mail. Share experiences that will create future memories: Do errands together, go on trips, and have coffee. Mostly, care about one another's lives and show up when needed.

Women's intimate relationships with their mates are not all they could be, according to recent research. A study published a few years ago in the *Journal of the American Medical Association* (*JAMA*) reported that a stunning 43 percent of American women are dissatisfied with their sex lives. According to the study, most of the sexual problems originated outside the bedroom door and were rooted in things such as anxiety, interpersonal problems, stress, and plain exhaustion.

If stress is the main stumbling block when it comes to making intimate sexual connections, try to think sexy when you're most rested, such as in the mornings and on vacation. Resist, though, the common prescription to schedule lovemaking into an already busy life. That makes it a duty, not a joy, and piles on performance pressure. Don't make dates for

> **Quick Tip:** *Get tuned in. Music can be a great stress reliever. A study at Ohio University, Athens, found that first-time blood donors who listened to music after donating were less likely to feel dizziness or nausea. Listen to instrumental music to relax, as it engages the right brain. Once you introduce lyrics, the left brain becomes involved and you start thinking about the words.*

10 ways to stress less and enjoy life more

1. *Surround yourself with positive people.* It's hard to stay miserable in a room full of optimists.

2. *Make a "happy list."* Even on your worst days, there are things you can appreciate at the moment.

3. *When facing a problem, don't sit around gloomily ruminating about it.* Instead, come up with three possible solutions. Chances are, one of them will solve your dilemma.

4. *Nourish your relationships by doing something small each day*—call a friend just to say hello; write a short love note to your mate; send a cartoon to a family member.

5. *Just do it.* If you've been putting off writing a short story or hiking the Appalachian Trail, what are you waiting for?

6. *Dance for joy.* Gyms are getting creative with classes such as Jock Ballet and bhangra, an Indian dance form. Or go out with your mate and swing or salsa dance.

7. *Do something you've never done before.* Paddle a canoe or go fishing.

8. *Find something to celebrate every month:* the change of seasons, the new moon, a "between" anniversary.

9. *Get near water as much as possible.* You'll find it calming in all its forms. Sit on a beach, by a river or lake, or get a tabletop fountain.

10. *Ask your partner what he really wants from you:* more communication, time alone together; evenings out? We often give important people in our lives what we want, so you may be surprised.

black sheep blues

Going against the family grain and not being understood by your relatives can be stressful. You get labeled the odd one out or the black sheep. But that can be a healthy thing. Choosing a path or lifestyle that's different from your family's "reflects your autonomy and independence," says Renee A. Cohen, Ph.D., a Los Angeles-based clinical psychologist who specializes in family therapy. You've learned to follow what's in your best interest instead of letting yourself be guided by other's wishes. On the other hand, maintaining relationships with people who question or disapprove of your choices can be stressful.

Don't explain your choices. Cohen points out that constantly defending yourself only gets you tangled up in more arguments. "The more you explain, the more material you give them to rebut," she says. Instead, focus on what you have in common. By concentrating on the things you share—history, common spiritual beliefs, and political values—and by inviting your relatives to occasionally share in your new experiences, you'll remind them that whatever your choices, they will still be family.

You can also "adopt" a family of your own. Whether it's a professional organization or a group of friends who share your personal beliefs, finding a community of like-minded people can provide a sense of support. Of course, most of us will form a "real" family of our own when we settle with a partner and have children. And according to the American Psychological Association guidelines for a strong, healthy relationship, breaking away from the birth family and establishing a new firm bond with your mate is key.

sex, make dates for pleasure: a gourmet picnic, a concert, a bike ride together, watching a sexy movie, or massaging each other. Good times together can strengthen your intimacy and consequently help improve your sexual connection.

Also, don't get stressed by movies or magazines that make a relationship filled with anything less then daily, mind-blowing sex seem dysfunctional. This is real life, and almost no one has a consistently perfect love life.

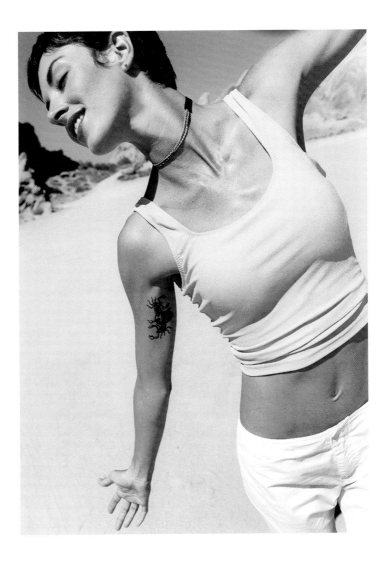

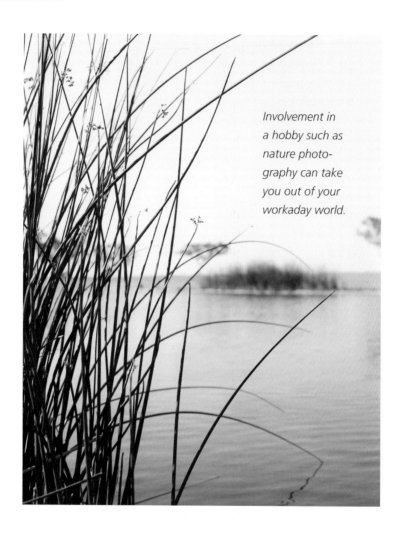

Involvement in a hobby such as nature photography can take you out of your workaday world.

pursue your passions

Sometimes stress comes from being in a rut: having too little rather than too much going on in your life. Ask yourself what's missing. With work and family monopolizing so much of your time, it could be that what you lack is fun, friends, and stimulation. You can often fill the missing pieces by pursuing an unfulfilled interest. Remember hobbies? The word calls to mind stamp albums, coin collections, and model airplanes built with glue and balsa wood. But hobbies aren't just kid stuff. Research shows that the passionate pursuit of our interests actually makes us happier and healthier.

Shape® reader Jessica Kaufman of San Francisco is a freelance photographer, but her real enthusiasm is reserved for an off-duty activity: rock climbing. "When I'm climbing, I'm totally engrossed in it," she says. "I don't think of anything else." Since she started her twice-weekly climbs, she's met like-minded friends and says she's a much happier person.

Experts say her experience isn't unusual: Serious hobbyists feel less anxiety, depression, and hostility, and enjoy more positive moods than people who spend their time in other ways. But how do these seemingly trivial pursuits make such a significant difference?

According to Douglas Kleiber, Ph.D., a University of Georgia professor and author of *Leisure Experience and Human Development,* hobbies are just plain fun. "Deep involvement in an activity can bring you great pleasure and joy," he says. Hobbies relieve stress, too, taking our minds off a troubled relationship or a hard day at work. They give us a gratifying sense of control: We can't dictate our boss's mood or our mate's schedule, but we can decide which trail to hike or which piano sonata to play. And when we do well by reaching the top of the mountain or mastering that tricky melody, we feel good about ourselves and our abilities.

Hobbies also offer a chance to try new things and learn new skills. "Leisure activities give you the freedom to explore other sides of yourself, develop other parts of your personality," says Kleiber. If you're impeccably organized and conscientious at work, you can use your after-hours interests to cut loose, painting a wild abstract canvas or riding your mountain bike through the mud. On top of everything else, sociable hobbies can bring you new friends, and sporty ones can help you get fit.

There's one catch: Only "serious leisure" offers all these benefits, according to Robert Stebbins, Ph.D., faculty professor of sociology at the University of Calgary in Canada. "Climbing mountains or playing the violin is serious leisure," he says. "Watching TV or sitting on a bar stool is not." Hobbies should be challenging enough to keep you interested, but not so difficult that you give up in frustration. And they should match up with your own tastes and inclinations. If you're a late riser who hates team sports, the early-morning soccer games will quickly lose their allure. Bottom line: Passion must be a key ingredient.

If you're not yet among the 20 percent of Americans who are avid hobbyists, it's never too late. "People with serious hobbies are no different from others in terms of their temperament or personality." Stebbins says. "They were just fortunate enough to have discovered something they enjoyed, and got hooked."

Follow our four-week plan to discover your passion:

Week One:

Look to your childhood for inspiration. Many of us have burrowed so deep into our daily routines that we've actually forgotten what it is we like to do. One way to recapture those lost interests is to reach back into our early memories. Get out some family photographs or home movies and take a look at yourself having fun. Talk to family members and old friends and reminisce about how you used to love spending afternoons and weekends as kids.

You can use those old favorites as a guide to activities you'd appreciate now. If your hands were always smeared with finger paint, for example, you'd probably take pleasure in a painting or sculpturing class. If nothing could keep you inside on a sunny day, joining a hiking club might satisfy your forgotten love of the outdoors.

Week Two:

Now look to your present life and decide what frustrates or excites you about it. Do you crave solitude and quiet time? Do group dynamics energize you? Is your job sedentary? Do you need more intellectual stimulation? The right leisure pastime can fill in the blanks.

Also examine whether the pleasure you get out of certain activities is "content- or context-based," says Richard Chang, Ph.D., author of *The Passion Plan: A Step-by-Step Guide to Discovering, Developing, and Living Your Passion*. When you engage in some specialized activity—swimming, dancing, cooking, playing a musical instrument, fishing—purely for the joy of it, then your passion is content-based. You don't care if you win, get paid, or have an audience. When you're inspired more by winning, creating, learning, leading, and helping others, then your passion is context-based. You'll likely get a kick out of competing or teaching a class, regardless of the particular activity involved.

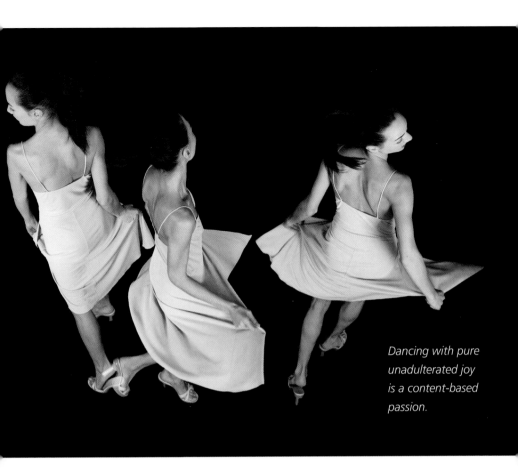

Dancing with pure unadulterated joy is a content-based passion.

Week Three:

By now you have an idea of what excites you, and what form your involvement might take. So this week start collecting information on how best to get started in your community. Say, for instance, that you were fascinated by bugs as a kid, would like more contact with people, and get a charge out of teaching: You might call your local natural history museum and see if they have a docent training program.

Check your Yellow Pages, library, hobby shops, and the Internet to locate clubs and interest groups in your area. You'll find that everyone from bead-jewelry makers to hang-gliding enthusiasts have their own associations. Your local university or community college will have not-for-credit classes in subjects you might not even have thought about—anyone for Japanese bookbinding or belly dancing? Many hobbies and sports also have their own magazines, and they're great resources on how to get started.

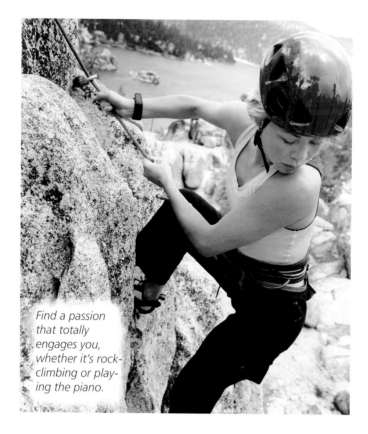

Find a passion that totally engages you, whether it's rock-climbing or playing the piano.

Week Four:

Try out some activities, with *try* being the operative word: Don't sign up for a lengthy course of classes or rush out and buy expensive equipment in a fit of enthusiasm. Sometimes just the newness of an activity will engage you initially, but then your interest might wane. Then what are you going to do with that $800 dressage saddle?

Once you've tried some activities, ask yourself these questions before committing more time and money:

- Do I lose track of time when I'm doing this activity?

- Do I feel energized afterward, even if I'm physically tired?

- Do I perform well and feel confident when I'm doing it?

- Can I hardly wait to do it again?

- Will this engage me in the long term?

- Does this fulfill my needs?

get beyond fear

We like to think of ourselves as daring and fearless: free to take up some exciting hobby such as skydiving or mountain climbing. But sometimes we can be held back from trying new things that will stimulate us or make us happy by fears and phobias. About 6.3 million Americans aged 18 to 54 suffer from some kind of phobia, says the National Institute of Mental Health (NIMH). The NIMH defines a phobia as an intense, illogical fear of a particular object or situation. Common sources of phobias include dogs, closed-in spaces, heights, escalators, tunnels, highway driving, and flying. Those fears certainly could curb the scope of your pleasurable activities.

Behavioral therapy can often help you figure out what's behind your panic and begin to deconstruct your phobia. But there are other strategies you can employ to help you overcome your fears, according to Alice Domar, Ph.D., director of the women's health programs at Harvard Medical School's Division of Behavioral Medicine.

Admit there's a problem. Don't underplay your fears or avoid discussing them because you're ashamed. "It's embarrassing to be afraid of something that most people don't think is frightening," says Domar. Once you admit your fear—to yourself and to others—you can start working toward getting over it.

Phobias are rooted in the unknown. Educate yourself. Often, people who are afraid to fly don't know how a plane stays in the air, or they think that planes crash more than they do. Although accidents and fatalities are quite rare, millions of American women are so crippled by this fear that they sacrifice the pleasures of foreign travel. According to an extensive study conducted by the Boeing Company, 18 percent of people surveyed were afraid of flying, and a further 12 percent expressed some anxiety about it. Another study by International Research Associates revealed that twice as many women as men were afraid of flying.

Be aware of your body. Fear causes physiological changes: Your heart races, and your breathing becomes shallow and rapid. Most people don't notice these physical symptoms when they're in panic mode. If you pay attention, you'll be able to keep them from taking control. By breathing slowly and deeply (inhaling from your belly, not your chest), your heart rate will slow and you'll think more clearly, helping to stem the panic.

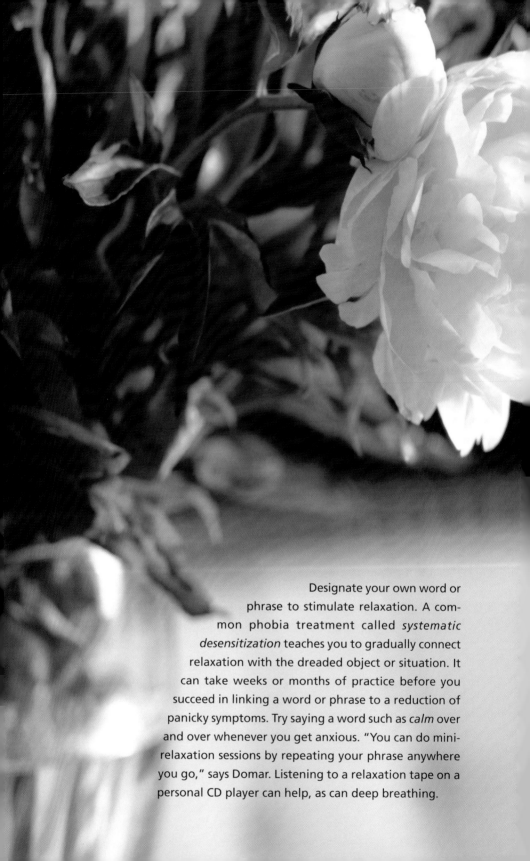

Designate your own word or phrase to stimulate relaxation. A common phobia treatment called *systematic desensitization* teaches you to gradually connect relaxation with the dreaded object or situation. It can take weeks or months of practice before you succeed in linking a word or phrase to a reduction of panicky symptoms. Try saying a word such as *calm* over and over whenever you get anxious. "You can do mini-relaxation sessions by repeating your phrase anywhere you go," says Domar. Listening to a relaxation tape on a personal CD player can help, as can deep breathing.

how to gain courage to try new things

With all of today's innovative fitness options, from flying-trapeze work-outs to surfing clinics, the problem isn't finding something new to try, it's getting up the nerve to go for it. Kate Hays, Ph.D., a sports psy-chologist, and founder of The Performing Edge in Toronto, offers some advice for visualizing and learning a new activity:

1. *Identify your motives.* Do you want to be able to join friends on weekend hikes, or to feel toned and confident in your bikini? "After pinpointing positive reasons for your new activity, you'll be able to think of it as an exciting adventure rather than something forced on you by yourself or others," says Hays.

2. *Give yourself a break.* "As adults, we're so used to being capable and successful that we forget what it's like to learn something new," says Hays. Remember that it's okay to be a beginner, and get comfortable with the idea that you might feel a bit uneasy at first.

3. *Be prepared.* Gather as much information as you can so you know what to expect. Hays suggests observing a class, checking out Websites where pros share tips, or posting a question on a message board. Also, enthusiasts often work in sporting goods stores and can answer questions.

4. *Shop around.* "It takes a special talent to know how to teach adult beginners," says Hays. Would you be more comfortable in a women-only environment, or maybe with someone you know? "Sometimes it's wonderful to be taught by a friend," says Hays. "But other times, it's more helpful to be taught by someone you have no connection with. Then you don't feel you need to please them."

just a habit

Habits are like the little girl with the curl in the middle of her forehead: when they're good, they're very, very good; when they're bad, they're horrid. Positive habits make us feel strong and virtuous; negative ones can make us feel weak and full of self-loathing.

Sure, we would all be fit, healthy, and energetic if only we could get into the habits of exercising regularly and eating only nutritious food, and break the routine of downing a pint of rocky road in front of the television every night. And it's not just the big habits that chip away at our health and cause stress. Your "harmless" habits—working long hours, eating on the run, staying up past bedtime—are just as insidious.

Chances are, you could probably name quite a few behaviors you'd like to change. So it's little wonder that so many of our self-improvement resolutions center on breaking habits. Yet even when we have the best intentions in the world, our resolutions are often circling the drain two weeks later, as we lapse back into ingrained patterns of behavior.

Why is it so difficult to cultivate new good habits and break old, bad ones? Roger Walsh, M.D., Ph.D., a professor of psychiatry, philosophy, and anthropology at the University of California at Irvine, says, "Humans were designed to habituate. Our brains are wired that way." It's habitual behaviors such as eating and sleeping, after all, that keep humans surviving as a species.

While those behaviors are instinctual, most of our habits are learned, often in childhood and from repetition. It's been said that a habit is like a sheet of paper: Once it's been creased, it tends to always fall into the same

> **Mistake to Avoid:**
>
> *Don't dwell on negative minutiae and overlook the positive big picture. For instance, you're at a friend's wedding— a glorious celebration— but all you can think about is how you look with the three pounds you've gained.*

fold. But even if your habits are as plentiful as folds in a road map, you can learn new ones.

Just don't attempt to change all your habits at once. A grand scheme to quit smoking, drinking, eating junk food, and being a couch potato simultaneously is likely to doom your efforts to failure. Pick one habit and focus on it. Decide which will be most encouraging to you: to master the hardest or the easiest one first. When the new health habit is entrenched, tackle the next one. And be specific: Instead of saying that you vow to eat better, determine to have a well-balanced breakfast while you make menu plans for the coming week.

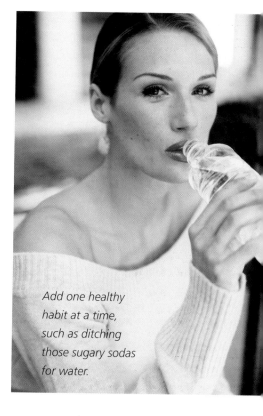

Add one healthy habit at a time, such as ditching those sugary sodas for water.

When embarking on a lifestyle change, the first thing you need to do is arrange your environment to support your desired new habit and remove sources of temptation that help perpetuate the old one. Say you're trying to quit eating so much ice cream—well, don't keep any in the freezer. (This might be difficult if your roommate, spouse, or kids still want their treats. Perhaps you could persuade them to go out for ice cream while you exercise or meditate.)

Announce your intentions to friends and family, and ask for their support. But if you suspect that they might not bolster your efforts or even sabotage them, keep your plans to yourself. You might want to "bribe" yourself or set up a system of healthful rewards. The idea is to do whatever it takes to stack the odds in your favor.

You'll also have to accept the need to be staunchly resolute until you've established your desired new habit. "Make no exceptions for the first month," says Walsh. It's tempting to convince yourself that just one cookie or just one missed workout session doesn't count. Psychologists say that "just one" is like dropping a ball of yarn you're trying to wind: It quickly unravels and runs out of control. Only once you no longer crave cookies is it safe to indulge in an occasional treat.

It isn't the act of starting a habit that counts, it's keeping it up. Doing something new can be hard at first, but with repetition it becomes easier, and eventually, automatic. As a bonus, you'll likely reach a point when you realize that this new activity is no longer difficult—it's actually enjoyable. You now eagerly look forward to having some delicious, seasonal fruit for dessert instead of regarding it as a poor second choice to a candy bar.

Quick Tip: *Speak a stress-free language. People who handle stress well tend not to beat themselves up when things don't work out in their favor. So instead of using statements that catastrophize an incident, such as "I'm awful at tennis," say, "I need to work on my backhand." Rather than saying, "I really blew that presentation," say, "That was a tough group to engage."*

Changing habits isn't about total deprivation. Making substitutions can help you during this stage because many habits are attached to other activities—eating while studying, for example. You might be most inclined to slip when you find you can't concentrate on your books without snacking. So instead of trying to give up eating completely, switch from candy or corn chips to fruit or air-popped corn.

In the process of substituting one habit for another, you need to remain mindful. Although the goal of establishing new habits is for them to become automatic, while you're in the process of changing you need to think about them. It's when you're not paying attention that you're most likely to lapse.

The moment of waking up is a great time to reaffirm your resolution to change and dedicate your day to transforming your habits, Walsh says. Throughout the day, whenever temptations prod you to backslide—stop, relax, and center yourself with a few deep breaths. Consider the consequences of your actions, then do what you know is best for you. Do something every day to reinforce your new habits. Having good intentions is only the beginning.

changing habits little by little

Kaizen (pronounced KI-zen) is an ancient Japanese Zen philosophy that advocates using "small, trivial steps to accomplish large goals," says Robert Maurer, Ph.D., faculty member of the UCLA School of Medicine. Although it may sound arcane, kaizen can be a valuable tool that anyone can use to change habits. The idea is to identify something you want to change, then break it down into steps so small that they appear to require little or no effort—for example, meditate for one minute, or drink one extra glass of water a day. "Doing this will get you in the right frame of mind, and the brain and body will begin to develop the habit," says Maurer. It's the tortoise-and-the-hare model of transformation: Small, deliberate steps can often get you to your goal quicker than if you sprinted and fell by the wayside.

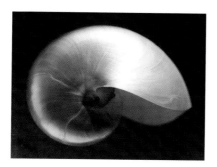

the program in action

Joanne Hewat had her first panic attack when she was on her honeymoon. One minute she was having a great time with her new husband, and the next she was consumed with uncontrollable fear. "My heart was pounding, and I was breathing hard and fast," she says. Upon arriving home, she saw a psychologist who concluded that the stress of planning the wedding, moving, and adjusting to married life was the culprit. She recommended stress-reducing activities such as exercise.

"Unfortunately," says Hewat, "I didn't take her advice and handled my stress by isolating myself from members of my family and many of my friends." Over the next three years, the attacks became worse, and Hewat spent her time at home cooking rich, high-fat foods that she ate herself. She gained 35 pounds, and that led to depression. Eventually, her marriage was affected by her panic attacks and depression, and she divorced.

She spent three years in this vicious cycle of overeating, depression, and isolation. Then she met the man who was to become her second husband. He suggested that they join a gym, and "although my workouts weren't very intense—usually just walking on the treadmill—I felt 100 percent better and my anxiety decreased," says Hewat. Soon, she moved on to aerobics classes and after six months had lost 15 pounds. After consulting a nutritionist, she also switched to healthy eating habits and immediately had more energy. She then lost ten more pounds.

"I haven't had a panic attack in years," says Hewat. "If I feel like I'm going to have an attack, I take my dogs for a walk, do yoga, or anything else to relax. I live a productive and fulfilling life, and family and friends are a regular part of my world. I'm finally in control of my mind and body, and life has never been better."

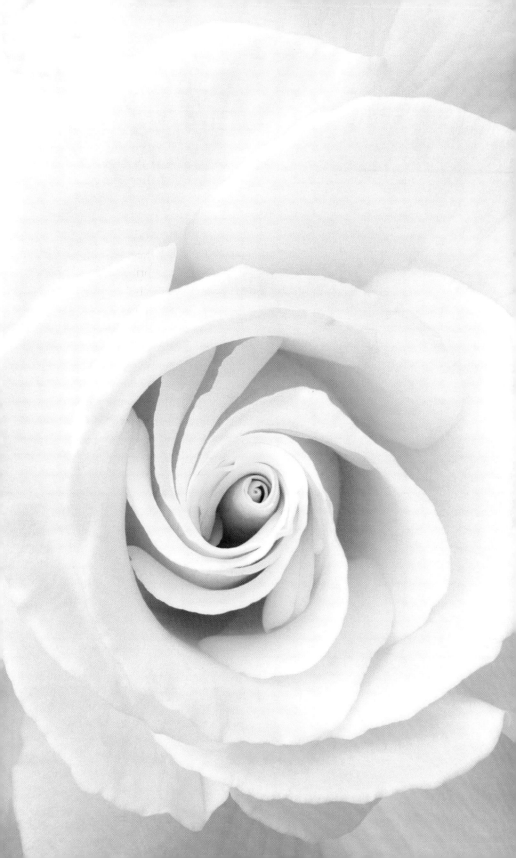

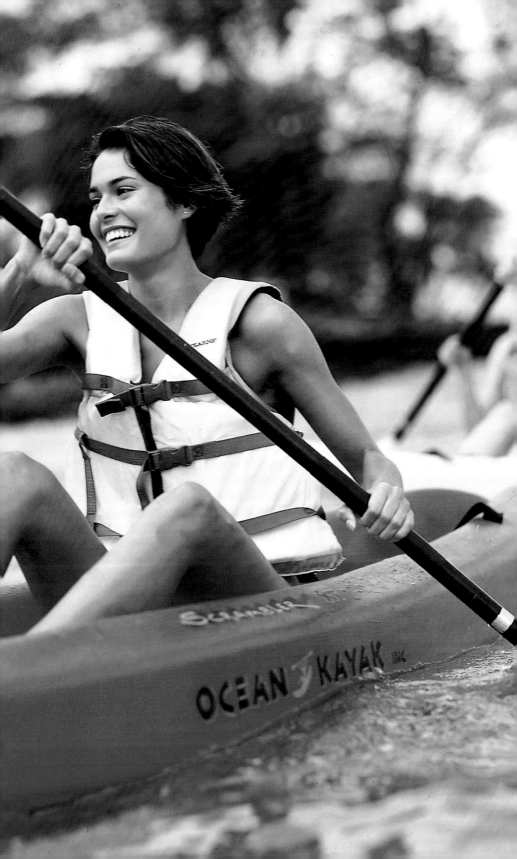

your body image

what you'll learn

Shape's approach to body image is that many women have a negative view of their bodies, and this is related to low self-esteem and self-consciousness. Using this chapter, you'll:

- get to the root of body-image issues
- build a positive view of your body at any size or shape
- counter "emotional eating"
- awaken to your physical nature
- formulate realistic goals

Mistake to Avoid:

Don't assume you'd be happier if you were just a little prettier. Researchers at York University in Toronto studied 203 women and found that the higher a woman was rated on a facial-attractiveness scale, the more likely she was to be unhappy with her weight. This dissatisfaction may increase the risk of developing eating disorders. To improve self-esteem, the study's author suggests focusing on non-appearance-related qualities, such as social skills and academic and athletic achievement.

how you'll do it

Do you have that constant negative hum in your head: "I'm too much of this . . . too little of that. . . ."? Do you compare your physical self with other women to decide if you like yourself? Do you like your body this year, but last year you could barely look at it? Or vice versa?

Maybe you answered, "All of the above." Our culture has a narrow definition of beauty exemplified by the runway model—tall and underweight, averaging 5'9" and 123 pounds. Where does that leave the majority of us—who average 5'4" and 144 pounds? For all too many of us, it leaves us with eating disorders, various levels of depression, and low self-esteem.

The topic has become the focus of serious attention among health professionals in recent years, and with good reason: The statistics are shocking. The National Association of Anorexia Nervosa and Associated Disorders (ANAD) reports that eating disorders have reached epidemic levels, and no segment of society or ethnic group is excluded. A reported seven million women are affected, and 86 percent of them say that the onset of the illness occurred before they turned 20. It's no wonder, really, since girls are dieting earlier and earlier, and reports of eating disorders have increased dramatically on college campuses. According to the ANAD, school and college programs addressing the dangers of eating disorders are practically nonexistent.

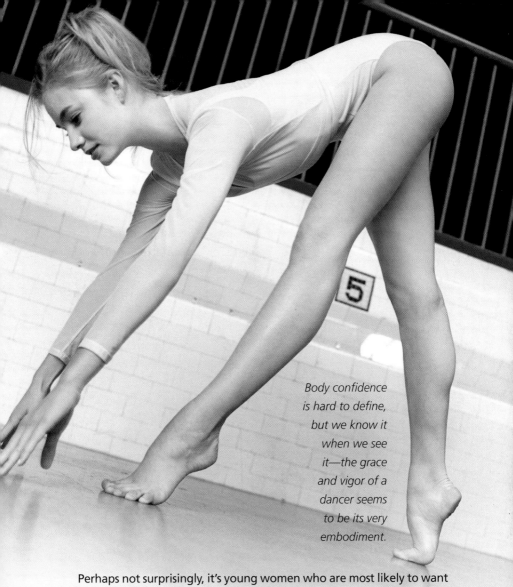

Body confidence is hard to define, but we know it when we see it—the grace and vigor of a dancer seems to be its very embodiment.

Perhaps not surprisingly, it's young women who are most likely to want to be thin, or at least thinner than they think they are. In an effort to recruit overweight college students for her weight-control course, Carol Kennedy, M.S., program director of fitness/wellness at Indiana University in Bloomington, offered a free body-fat percentage test to students as an incentive. What she found shocked her. "Seventy percent of the women who came in were in the normal range (20–30 percent body fat), but 56 percent perceived themselves as overweight," says Kennedy. She and her colleagues added a body-image class just for these women.

Of course, it's not just college-age women who have body issues. Women in their 20s and 30s contend with pressures of family, social, and

your body image

do you have a healthy body image?

Your attitude toward your body could be preventing you from enjoying the full and active life you deserve. Take our quiz to see how much you're held back by the tyranny of poor body image.

YES NO

___ ___ 1. I see my body as something that I need to fix.

___ ___ 2. My goals for my body are controlling my life.

___ ___ 3. I aspire to look like someone else.

___ ___ 4. I berate myself if I backslide.

___ ___ 5. I worry about how I appear to others.

___ ___ 6. I define success in terms of appearance.

___ ___ 7. I'm a slave to the scale and the mirror.

___ ___ 8. I deprive myself of pleasurable activity because of my appearance.

___ ___ 9. I look at my body reproachfully rather than appreciatively.

___ ___ 10. I frequently indulge in negative self-talk about my body.

SCORING

If you answered *yes* to even one of these questions, you may need to refocus your thinking and your goals. The path to authenticity begins with an honest appreciation of *your* body, with all of its strengths and vulnerabilities. Having unrealistic expectations of how your body should be—trying to manage it with weight control, clothing, and cosmetics, and aiming for others' idea of perfection when you haven't yet found self-acceptance—can all lead to frustration and a weak sense of identity.

working life; competition with peers; and nagging feelings of never quite being good enough, smart enough, or thin enough. Those in their 40s and beyond have to struggle with acceptance of the visible effects of aging in a youth-oriented society.

The American Society of Plastic Surgeons boasts that the number of people opting to surgically alter their bodies has tripled in the last ten years. The most requested procedure is breast augmentation, which has gone up by a whopping 533 percent, closely followed by liposuction, which has increased by 313 percent. The use of Botox for smoothing facial lines has exploded since it was given the green light for cosmetic use by the FDA, with "Botox parties" becoming a fad in some areas. Some shopping malls even have drop-in Botox shops.

"Women are more dissatisfied with their bodies today than ever before," says Sharlene Hesse-Biber, Ph.D., author of *Am I Thin Enough Yet?* The evidence is the women standing around the edges of the dance floor, both in a real and metaphorical sense—women who think they're too heavy or too unattractive to join in the fun. What they're actually lacking is body confidence.

body confidence

So what is body confidence, and where does it come from? It starts, say experts, with the role we expect the body to play. Is it active—a living being that moves and feels—or is it passive, an object to be looked at? To see body confidence in action, look no further than women athletes or dancers. In fact, engaging in sports or any physical activity is an excellent way to begin thinking of your body as active and, thus, not an object, says Elissa Koff, Ph.D., a psychologist and Wellesley College professor. "If you can feel like you're actually accomplishing something with your body, then you can shift the focus from the appearance of your body to the way your body operates in the world," says Koff.

A similar shift—this time from concerns about weight to concerns about health—is also crucial to body confidence. A diet and exercise program that's geared toward getting thin will only make you more conscious of the pounds you're trying to lose. But one that's aimed at achieving all-around good health and fitness—that is, what you can do with your

are you self-conscious during sex?

Regardless of whether they're thin or overweight, a third of young women worry about their appearance during sex, according to a survey of more than 200 college women published in *The Journal of Sex Research*. Such body-image anxiety can result in less satisfying sex, and in some cases, avoiding physical intimacy completely, say researchers. Women who feel the most self-conscious may be victims

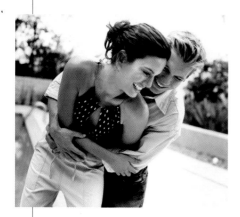

of those unrealistic cultural standards for female beauty and sex appeal. Fight-back strategies you can work on: Try to appreciate all sizes and shapes of bodies, including your own, and resist the urge to darken the room totally and hide yourself under the covers. And bear in mind, you're probably more critical of your body than your partner is.

body—will offer rewards well beyond a flat stomach or muscled biceps. "Even if you don't look the way you want to right away, healthy eating and exercise will make you feel better about life in general," says Yale psychologist and weight-issues expert Kelly Brownell, Ph.D. "You'll have more energy, you'll sleep better, your mood will improve." And research studies show that a lighter mood means that you'll be less critical of your body.

Accepting your body as it is represents another aspect of body confidence, one that begins with an awareness of your limits. "How you look is only partially under your control," Brownell reminds us. "People assume that appearance is entirely driven by personal behavior, but that's not so." Learning to accept your physical inheritance is an integral part of good body image. So is the strength to resist unrealistic standards of beauty imposed from the outside. Women with body confidence appreciate the natural variation in the bodies of the women they see around them.

A generous attitude toward other women, in fact, is another foundation of body confidence because competition and comparison only worsen insecurities all around.

In the end, body confidence is not really about your physical form. It's about your life and how you live it. As Brownell notes, "So many people say, 'When I lose weight I will . . .' then fill in the blank: Get a new job. Leave a bad relationship. Move to another city." People with body confidence know that the time is *now,* whatever size they're wearing. They don't link their happiness to a number on the scale, and they don't let their bodies become lightning rods for negative feelings.

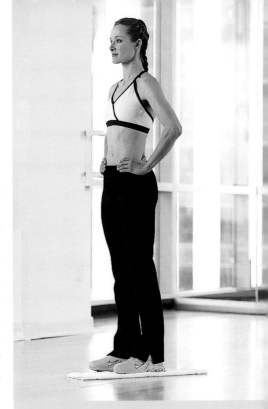

your mother, your body

When it comes to the source of our body image, often we blame Mom, her own body image, and the way she shaped our eating habits. Everyone has their own story about mothers and food. But in the last generation or so, the storyline has changed. It used to go something like this: *Eat your vegetables. Finish what's on your plate. Don't you want to grow big and strong? Why aren't you eating? Are you hungry?*

Quick Tip: *See yourself as you really are. When researchers at St. George's Hospital Medical School in London asked 50 women to estimate the width of a box, they were right on target. But when asked to estimate their own body size, they inflated the girth of their waists by about 25 percent and their hips by about 16 percent.*

Now the script is often closer to this: *Eat your vegetables* (no escaping that one). *Do you really want to eat that? Too many of those will make you fat. You know, bread has a lot of calories. Be careful—the women in our family have always been heavy.*

Mothers have always held powerful sway over their daughters' ideas about eating, and consequently, body image—after all, feeding their children has been their evolutionary duty for most of human history. The difference is that today's young adult women of childbearing years are the first to have grown up with mothers who themselves were raised in a thinness-obsessed, diet-crazed culture. The 1960s introduced super-thin, Twiggy-type models, weight-loss centers, and fad diets, and women's feelings about how to eat and look have not been the same since.

In fact, according to Debra Waterhouse, M.P.H., R.D., author of *Like Mother, Like Daughter: How Women Are Influenced by Their Mothers' Relationship with Food—and How to Break the Pattern,* we are now embarking on a third "dieting generation," and a frightening pattern is emerging. Each generation starts dieting at an earlier age. Consider, say, the case of a ten-year-old showing off her new bathing suit, and her mother reflexively saying, "Hold in your stomach." You can almost hear the words echoing down the years, until at age 25 the daughter sits in a body-image therapy session recounting how her mother made her feel fat.

> **Mistake to Avoid:**
>
> *Don't feel guilty if you're envious of friends' looks. Turn those feelings into motivation to make changes in your own life. When you find envy creeping up on you, do something to bring yourself closer to your goal—walk the stairs in you office building to boost your fitness, or write down why you deserve to feel great about your body.*

class act

Some life events trigger feelings of insecurity about our lives and looks. Class reunions are a perfect example. In a recent survey of more than 1,000 women, respondents said that the main topic of conversation after a reunion was "how people looked." So it's no surprise that panic can set in when one is looming on the horizon: "I've got to lose 25 pounds . . . I hate the way I look . . ." In fact, 33 percent of the women surveyed said that not being happy with their looks might be enough to keep them away from an upcoming reunion altogether.

"Class reunions are bookmarks in time that make us want to compare and compete with our peers," says Ellen McGrath, Ph.D., a clinical psychologist in New York. But instead of revamping everything about yourself, let reunions be a well-timed opportunity for self-assessment. "Rate how well you've been taking care of yourself, eating, and exercising," she says. Use it as a good reason to get a new haircut, to splurge on a new dress, or to hire a trainer or nutritionist—not to crash diet, exercise obsessively, or put yourself into credit-card debt overhauling your wardrobe. "Focus on all you have accomplished, experienced, and enjoyed over the past years," says McGrath, "and communicate that sense of confidence to your old classmates."

"Research has shown that one important way you develop body image is through identification with a same-sex parent," says Ann Kearney-Cooke, Ph.D., director of the Cincinnati Psychotherapy Institute, and an expert in body-image and eating disorders. Thus, logically, the mother who obsesses about her own thick waist or heavy thighs passes along a view of herself and the world: There's something wrong with you if you're not thin. Embedded in that message is also the idea that being thin will make a crucial difference in your quality of life.

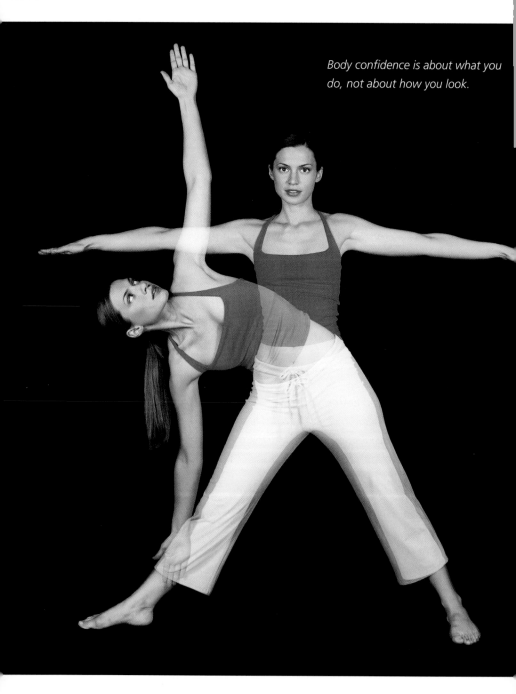

Body confidence is about what you do, not about how you look.

This transmission of values can happen in two different ways, according to Kearney-Cooke. One is the identification process, in which you indirectly absorb your mother's values and worldview even if she never directly comments on it. You watch her trying on ten outfits, none of which makes her feel attractive; you observe her ordering salads with dressing on the side, and chatting with friends about the latest diet. You understand quite clearly, and at a young age, that women restrict their food, often feel overweight and unattractive, and strive endlessly toward slenderness.

The second way is the internalization process, in which the message is more overt. People make comments to you about your eating and your body, and you take them in and make them part of your psyche—as the ten-year-old in the aforementioned example might do. "It's like being branded," Kearney-Cooke says. "Very often the comments come from people who are overly concerned with their own bodies, and they're extending that to their child." The mother of the young girl has likely repeated a litany to herself countless times: "Hold your stomach in."

Kearney-Cooke cites research indicating that when a mother is critical of her own body, she's more critical of her daughter's shape, and the daughter in turn tries to control her body in particularly destructive ways: extreme diets and eating disorders.

Without question, the mother-daughter connection is powerful and can be convoluted and, as we all know, often fraught with unstated conflict. A mother may feel jealous of the emerging beauty of her daughter, or may identify almost too strongly with her daughter—if her daughter is heavy, the mother may feel that it reflects on her in some negative way. A daughter may feel inadequate next to the all-powerful archetypal female exemplified by her mother, as if she will never measure up.

But there's good news here: Underlying these tensions there's typically great love and concern. Many mothers who try to influence their daughters' physical shape have learned firsthand the harsh reality that women are still judged by their appearance. Many meddling mothers are actually trying to smooth their daughters' way in the world. It's a fact in our culture today: Your life is harder if you don't conform to society's standards.

10 ways to boost your body image

1. *Try new activities to loosen up your inhibitions,* such as African, hula, or belly dancing.

2. *Use your body to do something*—build a shed, score a field goal, carry an elderly neighbor's groceries—instead of treating it as an object to be looked at.

3. *Get to know your body's abilities and limitations* through challenging physical activity: rock climbing, roller skating, diving, biking, windsurfing, scuba diving.

4. *Indulge your sensual side:* Get massages, use exotic perfumes, wear sexy lingerie (only *you* may know you're doing so, but you'll project a more confident face to the world).

5. *Wear clothes that allow you to move freely:* comfortable shoes, flowing skirts, stretchy fabrics. And don't worry about size, only about fit and how your clothes make you feel.

6. *Learn about the wonders of the female body:* Read *Woman: An Intimate Geography* by science writer Natalie Angier. Or get *really* intimate with it by reading *The Vagina Monologues* by Eve Ensler.

7. *Try yoga or meditation:* They're two good practices that teach you how to be in your body in a way that isn't critical or analytical.

8. *Get involved in a cause*—it will put things in perspective. You'll realize that in the big picture, how you look isn't that important.

9. *Practice good posture.* It's an instant shot of body confidence.

10. *Quit believing that people are looking at you and sizing you up.* Most of the time, they're thinking about themselves.

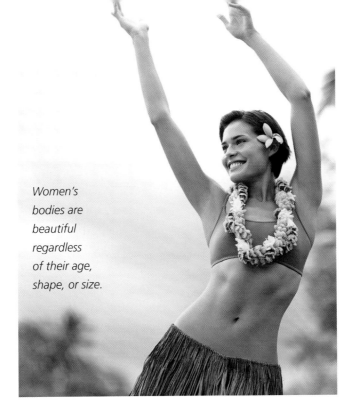

Women's bodies are beautiful regardless of their age, shape, or size.

the message in the media

If Mom sets the body-image ball rolling, popular culture keeps it in play. Impossibly thin models advertise almost every known product, while celebrities tell compelling stories about how they used to be 20 pounds "overweight"—just like you and me—until they whittled their waists, through diet and determination, into size-two jeans. Consequently, we force near-impossible expectations upon ourselves: Our jeans are in conflict with our genes.

"It's disturbing," says Cathy Conheim, LCSW, a co-founder of The Real Women Project, which uses the arts to broaden our society's definition of beauty and to deepen women's self-esteem and well-being. "We're addicted to images of women that are not about reality. We look at women in magazines, on television, and in movies and say, 'Well, I don't look like that, so there must be something wrong with me.'"

At the heart of the Real Women Project is a five-year traveling exhibit consisting of 13 small sculptures of nude women ranging from 14 to 75.

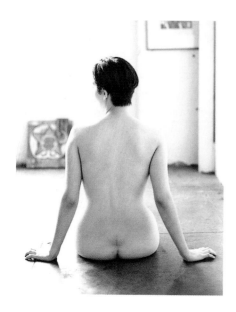

The message the project founders wanted to convey was that women's bodies are beautiful throughout the life cycle and beyond our culture's narrow definitions of beauty. Discovering themselves naked was transformative for the real women who were the models for the exhibition. "Until I was 33, when I posed for the sculpture," says Zona, one of the models, "I had not come to terms with my body. I live in Southern California where there's a lot of pressure to have a certain look. I think it's a travesty that women spend most of their sexual lives trying to look like someone else. Posing for the sculpture really made me begin to love my body and think positive thoughts about it. It really changed me."

Conheim contends that a key aspect of realistically assessing your own body is to get to know it naked. Few women spend enough time with themselves naked to be objective about their bodies, she says, and she recommends that we all try taking a good look at ourselves naked. All you need is you—and a private spot at home with a full-length mirror. Most of us will look in the mirror and judge ourselves severely. We'll suck in our guts. We'll wish the back view were smaller. We'll say, "If only my thighs or my hips weren't so big." You may have feelings ranging from sorrow to anger to vulnerability. "Negative feelings about your body may come up," says Conheim. "Explore where they come from, perhaps judgments from your family, an old boyfriend, or messages from the media and our culture."

Continue doing this until you learn to *describe* your body parts (for example, "my calves are muscular"), rather than *judge* them ("my calves are thick and ugly"). "Reality is wondrous," says Conheim. "We need to celebrate it, not run from it." She uses this technique in the body-image workshops she holds for women.

Shape®, too, holds body-image workshops, and psychologist Ann Kearney-Cooke, Ph.D., says that the group experience is powerful. It allows participants to discover together that body image is really much more about how satisfied you are with your life. "Every group I've been with goes through this same progression," she says. "Everyone thinks at first that it's about their weight, shape, how big their thighs are. What they learn is that the body is a screen on which they're projecting their lives—their relationships with other people, their feelings about themselves, their fears or feelings of shame. And they can't change their body images until they change what's going wrong with those other things in their lives." You'll find the body-image workshops powerful forums for transformation (see **Shape.com**).

Or, you can develop your own workshop to help you learn to live in your skin just a little differently. The idea is to get four to five friends together and begin a discussion group on how your ideas about your bodies were formed.

Conheim has formulated some questions for you to promote discussion that will challenge our culture's narrow definitions of beauty. Write the questions down and drop them into a hat. Each woman picks one question, reads it aloud, and then gets down to listening and sharing with the group. Since you won't have a group leader, we've also included some suggestions on how to use the answers the group comes up with.

Quick Tip: *In your interactions with friends, try to connect only with women who support and nurture the idea of inclusive beauty; avoid those who are critical or obsessed with weight. Make it clear that you're not interested in making judgments about other women's bodies, and no longer will you be engaging in put-downs or stereotyping.*

- **Question:** Which parts of your body do you like the most? How much time have you dwelled on them?

  Suggestion: You probably don't spend a lot of time dwelling on the things you love about yourself. Wake up each morning and take a minute to think about them.

- **Question:** Who in your life has made you feel most beautiful physically? How?

  Suggestion: Make sure you spend a little time each day remembering how good that felt. Try to recall that feeling when thoughts turn negative.

- **Question:** How much time have you spent thinking about changing aspects of your body? What do you imagine would be different in your life?

  Suggestion: Spend time thinking about how much you like certain aspects of your body and how you would never change them for a minute.

- **Question:** What are the three most important messages you remember your mother or father teaching you, through words or behavior, about your physical beauty? Are the messages healthy ones? Does this still affect you today?

  Suggestion: If the messages were negative, understand that your parents' messages may have been poorly expressed, and their true intention was for you to grow up healthy and happy. Forgive them, and take a realistic look at the part of you that felt attacked.

- **Question:** When in your life did you start comparing yourself to other women? Do the comparisons create positive or negative feelings?

  Suggestion: Take the judgment out of comparisons with other women. Say, "I'm different from her in this way," instead of "She looks better than I do because she is . . ."

- *Question*: If you had a daughter, how would you help her shape her concept of beauty?

  Suggestion: Make a point to purchase dolls for her in a variety of shapes, sizes, and colors. Read books to her that show many different ways of being successful. Show her magazines with photos of children of varying ethnicities. Talk to her frequently about the different aspects of beauty, both inner and outer.

Even if you can't, or don't want to, get a group together, there's much value in responding to the questions yourself. There are no right or wrong answers—the point is to find out what you really feel about your body, how you came to feel that way, and whether or not your beliefs about it are good for your emotional health. It's an exercise in becoming intimate with yourself, with the hope that you'll move further along in feeling good about your body just as it is—and begin to approach your health and fitness from a positive point of self-acceptance.

You can begin that exploration toward transforming your attitudes by following our four-week program. These exercises all involve listening to, and starting to change, your inner dialogues, with a view to ultimately changing the negative ways you think and feel about your body:

> **Quick Tip:** *According to the National Eating Disorders Association, people with a negative body image have a greater likelihood of developing an eating disorder. If you think you have anorexia or bulimia, get information and help from the association at (206) 382-3587 or* **www.nationaleatingdisorders.org.**

Week One:

This week, carefully listen to your own inner voice. We often "say" things to ourselves that we wouldn't say to—or accept from—others. Monitor your thoughts, and when they're needlessly negative, stop and ask yourself: "How much of this dialogue comes from my parents, my education, my culture, and my experiences? Whose values do I live? What influences have come together to form my view of myself? What are my true gifts and limitations?"

Journaling—writing down your thoughts and feelings—is a great way to help you find the answers. Just don't be discouraged if what you put down seems superficial or trite at first. "Keep writing until something happens," says Kearney-Cooke.

Week Two:

Work this week on banishing that internal voice—the anxious mother within—and replacing it with an accepting, centered voice: your own. "You may need to separate internally from your mother somewhat in order to challenge any distorted thinking you may have picked up from her," says Kearney-Cooke. "Step back and observe her more objectively if you can. Begin to understand where some of your attitudes come from. Then you have to say to yourself, 'I'm the author of my own story now.'" If you can't banish your mother's ingrained attitudes on your own, you may want to seek the help of a therapist or dietitian, who will help you create your own attitudes about food and your body.

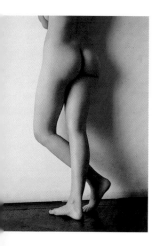

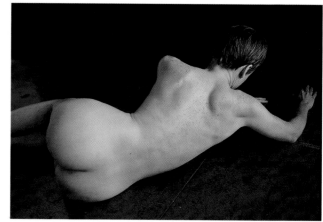

Week Three:

Start to change your body thoughts. Kearney-Cooke offers this parable to get you started: A polar bear is sent to a new zoo. He arrives early and must stay in a cage while his habitat is being finished. For a month, he paces the cage. At last, he's released into the expansive new environment, replete with pools, rocks, and new playmates. Yet he continues to walk in a square, mentally trapped in his pattern, unable to see that he's free.

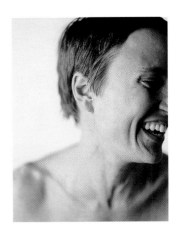

The moral is that you must think your way out of the cage you've constructed for yourself. When body-bashing hits this week, instead of just pacing those four corners of "I'm fat," "My thighs are huge," "I'm ugly," "I have no self-control," stop and ask: "What situation am I in right now? Who am I with? What else might be bothering me?" According to Kearney-Cooke, negative thoughts about one's body distract us from the really tough issues. It's easier to go with those familiar self-loathing themes than to think, for instance, about whether we're getting what we need from others, what we're afraid of, and what we're hungry for.

Week Four:

Now it's time to start allowing your authentic voice to be heard. To do that, plan for some quiet time. Don't feel compelled to cram every moment of your day with activities and external stimuli. Women often rely on staying busy to avoid feelings of self-hatred that arise when they're alone or bored. Similarly, don't try to assuage painful feelings of emptiness by filling yourself up with food. "Stay with the emptiness; it can take shape if you don't fill it," says Kearney-Cooke. Still your mind with practices such as meditation or quiet walks in nature, and listen for your deeper and truer voice to emerge.

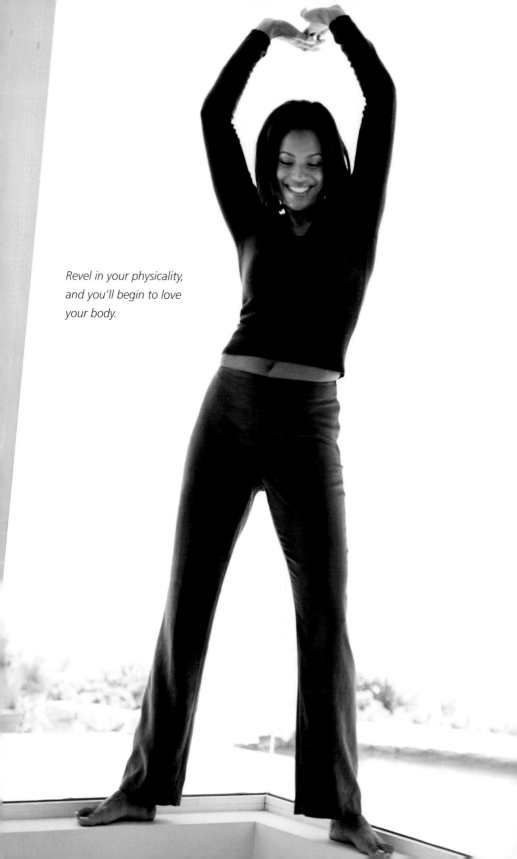

*Revel in your physicality,
and you'll begin to love
your body.*

exercise your option
for a better body image

There may be no magic bullet to make you love your body more, but getting healthy and strong by becoming active and taking good care of yourself comes close. The problem is that many women approach exercise and fitness with the wrong goal in mind.

When you ask women to define their fitness goals, most of us rattle off what we'd like to *lose:* weight, saddlebags, tummy bulge, back fat, cellulite. But ask what we'd like to *gain,* and many of us can't say for sure. We miss out with this approach because there's so much to be gained: the joy of transformation, the thrill of accomplishment, the pleasure of awakening to your physical nature, and the satisfaction of taking care of your body—including getting the rest you need and feeding your body healthfully.

Too often we force near-impossible expectations upon ourselves: to squeeze into a certain size or look like some TV star. And in doing so, we deny ourselves the pleasure of appreciating our bodies: as they are, what they actually can become, and the joy we can have in the moment.

It may be more effective for a woman who wants to shed pounds and inches to forget about weight loss as a goal. Action-based goals may be just what she needs to succeed. "Professional athletes approach goals from a performance angle, focusing on what they need to do," says James Loehr, Ed.D., president of LGE Performance Systems in Orlando, Florida. They don't judge effectiveness by standing in front of a mirror. When you're focused on achievement, and when you measure and meet performance-based goals in increments (such as walking an extra half mile, or increasing weight on your lat pull-downs), weight loss will take care of itself.

As you set specific, concrete exercise performance goals you can measure (maybe eventually you'd like to run a 10K, but today need to accomplish a mile, for example), you also learn to give your body what it needs to attain them. It feels good when you're building a body that's faster, stronger, and fitter. And with all the training, a skimpy green salad for dinner won't do.

"Health and nutrition are very much connected to performance," says Loehr. "If you do anything that jeopardizes your health, the whole thing comes apart." Achieving what you set out to do with your body begins with the first simple act of respecting it. Treat it well, mentally and physically, and it will reward you in return.

To get yourself oriented toward physical performance rather than appearance goals:

- Think differently. Don't visualize yourself as a sitting person— see yourself as a moving person.

- Define success in terms of what you accomplish daily. Is even climbing the stairs easier?

- Avoid the scale, especially if you've started weight training. It may lie about your progress.

- Don't measure success by looking in the mirror.

- Allow yourself setbacks. They're inevitable. Remember, you're in it for the long haul.

- Balance fitness goals with life goals. Define what you're excited about achieving in other areas of your life. Living a passionate life that brings you satisfaction can keep exercise and body-image goals in perspective.

So how do you set a long-term goal that goes beyond losing ten pounds? Think of challenges you've dreamed of meeting, and follow our four-week plan to get started. Within six months to a year, you may be running a 10K race or a marathon, cycling 100 miles, kayaking for a week among killer whales in British Columbia, or hiking the Appalachian Trail.

what's behind the "perfect" body?

When looking for healthy-body role models, you might have turned to the gym. You've probably asked your favorite exercise teacher how she keeps so toned and what eating regimen she follows. But she may not be the person to ask. A study conducted at Indiana University in Bloomington showed that despite having an average body-fat per-

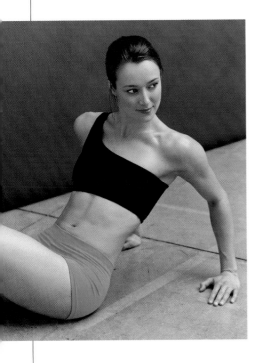

centage lower than most women their ages, 148 fitness instructors still wanted to be thinner and weren't happy with their figures. Findings revealed that no matter how great they look, fitness instructors are at a particularly high risk for eating disorders, pathological overexercising, and body-image disorders. The problem is, they're expected to be walking advertisements for their services. But you never know how someone achieves the perfection you see, and this is another reason not to idolize the "perfect body." Rather than choosing an instructor based solely on her appearance, find one who also offers sound ad-

vice. Try to determine whether this is a person who can help you reach realistic goals for a fit, healthy body through a reasonable time commitment and who also takes a holistic approach, balancing fitness goals with life goals. And look at the gym's other members for inspiration: "real" people of all types of body shape and size enjoying their workouts and getting healthy.

Week One:

Identify your natural abilities, and the activities that are best suited for your body, then come up with a physical challenge that's beyond what you're capable of doing now. Gather ideas by looking through adventure travel articles in past issues of *Shape®*, adventure-travel catalogs, and Websites including **ivillage.com, lonelyplanet.com, gorp.com,** or **adventurewomen.com**. You don't have to leave home, though. Look for events in your local area such as fund-raising races. Buy a journal, and use it to write down your goal and your motivation for wanting to engage in the activity. On another page, make a collage of what you imagine the experience will be like.

Week Two:

Find a trainer or coach to help you set up a training program. Plan necessary classes to help you achieve your goal, and record your progress in your journal. For example, if your goal is to kayak for a week with an adventure-travel company, take an introductory kayaking class through your local community college or outdoor adventure store. Even if the travel company provides instruction, you'll enjoy becoming familiar with the techniques before you go.

Week Three:

Begin keeping a training log. Break your training down into phases. You'll be recording your progress along the way in your journal. Among the things you'll note are your progress, how your body changes physically, and how you feel. Do you feel stronger? Can you do more sets and reps during weight training? Can you run the same distance more easily?

Week Four:

Now that you've started your training program, record your transformation in your journal. Include any mementos that motivate and inspire you, including photos. You could also do this on your computer, making a Website that charts your progress.

suit yourself

Is there any event more destined to send your self-image plummeting than trying on a new swimsuit in a store's fitting room? Those fluorescent lights . . . those judgmental salespeople . . . those three-way "fat" mirrors. . . . To take some of the sting out of the experience:

1. *Invest in some self-tanner.* Next time you see one of those before-and-after weight-loss ads, notice how when the pasty "before" woman morphs into her new, slim "after" self, she's sporting a St. Tropez tan. This is no coincidence. Just as dark colors hide a multitude of sins, properly applied self-tanner camouflages cellulite, spider veins, and uneven skin tone. Give yourself a week to get a golden tan-from-a-tube before even thinking about hitting the mall.

2. *Bring a friend.* Your friend won't snicker when you choose a large bottom and a small top. She wouldn't dream of suggesting that you pad your top with gelatinous inserts to "balance you out." And when you've had enough, she'll head for the java joint with you and laugh about this year's swimsuit fashions over a tall latte.

3. *Hit the gym.* No, one more step class won't launch your *Sports Illustrated* swimsuit career. What you're doing here is checking out the other women—everyone does it. By participating in this voyeuristic ritual, you're reminding yourself that real bodies come in an array of shapes and sizes, very few of them being Barbie-esque.

4. *Get over it.* Presumably, you're buying this suit in anticipation of some sort of fun in the sun. You're going to be playing volleyball, surfing, or snorkeling. Maybe you'll be sailing to exotic islands or donning your scuba gear and plumbing the depths of some remote ocean. Don't let your outfit dampen any great experience you have planned.

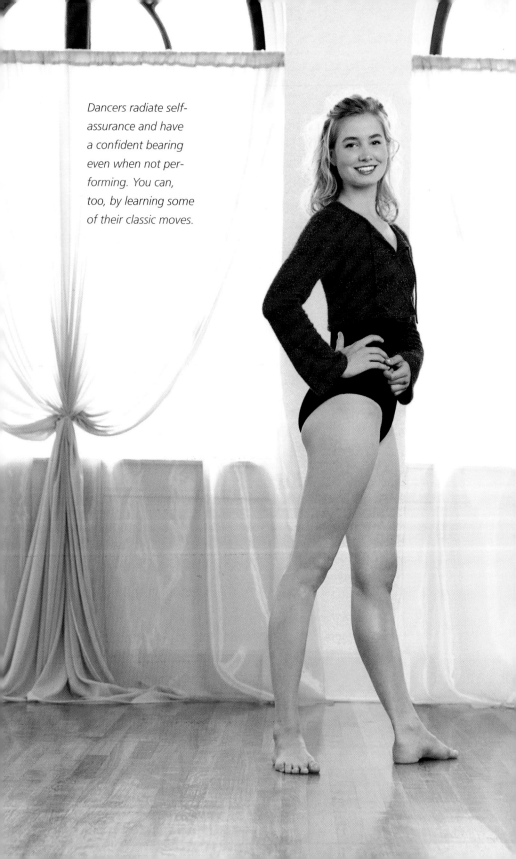

Dancers radiate self-assurance and have a confident bearing even when not performing. You can, too, by learning some of their classic moves.

the boost-your-body-image workout

Think about dancers—whether Vegas showgirls wearing 20 pounds of beads and feathers on their heads (and often little else!), funky hip-hop divas on MTV, or those Irish Riverdancers—they have one thing in common: supreme body confidence. Perhaps the most poised of all of them are ballet dancers.

"The fluid grace of a dancer comprises the complete mastery and balance of strength and flexibility," says Kari Anderson, a renowned dance exercise teacher and former professional dancer who teaches in Seattle. "But despite the physical exertion, they must make everything look effortless. They make their hard work look easy and beautiful."

A dancer's energy comes from her torso. Her abs, chest, back, pelvis, and buttocks radiate a feeling of strength, composure, and power all the way out to her limbs. In ballet, one leg is supporting the dancer's weight, while the other leg is working. You can spot real dancers by the way they hold themselves on the standing leg, rather than sinking their weight down on it. Aspiring ballerinas are taught to always think up, up, up, giving them a beautiful, confident-looking bearing.

While you may never leap across the floorboards of a Broadway theater, you can help achieve the posture, carriage, and joyful energy of a dancer with the four ballet exercises designed by Anderson. All you need is a counter or chair back for support. Choose a quiet place that encourages you to breathe deeply, and focus on how your body is moving as well how it feels. When you do the moves, don't worry about how high you lift your leg. Instead, concentrate on keeping your body in alignment: pelvis stable, limbs long, and abdominal muscles engaged. (Oh, yes, you'll also get a great leg and buttocks workout, too.)

To get even more into dance exercise, check out Anderson's videos, available from Great Moves Video: (206) 729-0365 • *e-mail:* greatmovesvideo@aol.com.

the plan

Do the workout 3 times a week as part of a program that includes upper-body strength moves and cardio.

Week One: Do 1 set of 10 reps for each exercise.
Week Two: Do 2 sets of 10 reps each.
Week Three: Do 3 sets of 10 reps each.
Week Four: Start to increase the reps, working up to 15.

Warm up by freestyle dancing to music you like for 5–10 minutes, then do some gentle stretching. Cool down with more freestyle dancing and stretching that focuses on the hips and lower body.

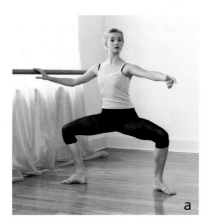 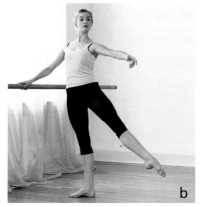

a · b

1. Grand Plié with Leg Lift. *Stand in second position: legs rotated out from the hips and toes pointing out, right hand on chair back or support, left hand held softly out from the shoulder, head looking to the left; elbow and wrist curved. Slowly bend knees into a grand plié, thighs approaching parallel to floor, knees centered over toes (a). Using your glutes and thighs and pressing heels into floor, push up. Near the top of the move, shift your weight to your right leg, and lift the left leg off floor in a straight line (b). Place left foot back on floor, descend into another grand plié, and repeat 10 times. Switch sides and repeat.*
   Works hamstrings, quadriceps, and gluteals.

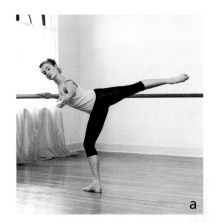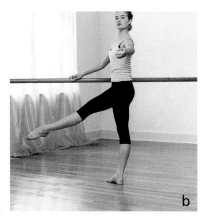

2. Arabesque and Leg Swing. *Stand in first position: heels together, hips comfortably rotated out, toes pointing out, torso lifted, right hand on the chair back or support, and left arm as in move #1. Keeping thighs rotated out, use glutes to brush left leg back, allowing torso to move forward and down until torso and leg are in one line (flat-back arabesque). Keep head in line with spine looking out over left arm (a). Bring leg back to first position and torso to vertical, then brush leg forward, approaching hip height. Stop when you can no longer maintain turnout (b). Return to first position and repeat 10 times. Switch sides and repeat.*

    Works hamstrings, quadriceps, gluteals, and adductors.

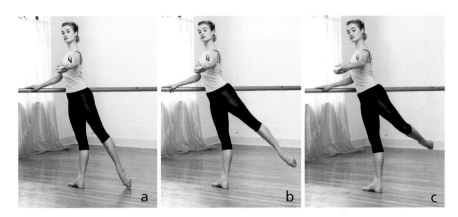

3. Tendu to Attitude Lift. *With feet in first position (see move #2), right hand on the chair back, left arm in second position (held softly out from the shoulder), brush your left leg behind you until just the side of the big toe is on the floor (tendu) (a). Use glutes to slowly lift the leg off the floor to a height you can maintain; continue rotating out from the hips (arabesque) (b). Keeping abs tight, bend left knee, bringing left foot behind right leg without moving hips (back attitude) (c). Tighten glutes and hold for a moment, then bring leg back to (b) position for one count. Return to (a) position. Do 10 reps, then switch sides and repeat.*
    Works gluteals, adductors, abductors, and quadriceps.

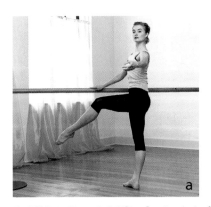
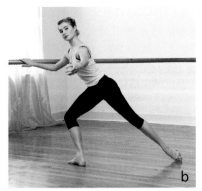

4. Plié to Front Attitude. *Begin in first position, right hand on chair back, left arm in second position. Keeping torso lifted, brush left leg back to tendu. Maintaining hip rotation, slowly bend standing leg into a plié, keeping left leg straight while sliding toes behind you (on floor) until you form a straight line from top of head to foot (a). Using glutes and thigh muscles and keeping abs tight, straighten standing knee and slide toes back to first position. Continue rotating from hips, and brush leg forward to hip height, bending knee and trying to keep heel high (front attitude) (b). Return to first position. Do 10 reps, then switch sides and repeat.*
    Works gluteals and adductors.

the program in action

Dawn Basham's childhood dream was to become an actress and a singer, so when she was accepted to a prestigious performing arts school in New York City, she was ecstatic. But during her first year, she felt lonely and became depressed. "I started drinking, smoking, and eating to make myself feel better," she says. "Although it perked me up for a while, in the end I felt worse. I gained weight and felt helpless as the pounds piled on." By the time she graduated, she'd gained 30 pounds.

Then came the tough part: going before casting directors for acting jobs. "I went on a couple of auditions," she says, "but they were disastrous since I felt uncomfortable and self-conscious in my body." Slowly she stopped trying and began earning a living as a waitress. As months passed, she realized that her dream was slipping away, and she became determined to make changes.

First she quit smoking cold turkey—"one of the hardest things I ever did." Then she went to a counselor to deal with her depression. As part of her treatment, her therapist suggested that she join a gym and start weight training, since it would boost her self-image. "I was skeptical at first," says Basham, "but amazingly, she was right. I started lifting weights every other day and walking." She shed the fat from her body and developed lean, beautiful muscles. Whenever she felt depressed, Basham would challenge herself to walk, swim, or do any other activity that she knew would make her feel better about herself.

She has maintained her healthy mind-set for three years now, and "it's part of my life, like breathing." She's now working as a model, singer, and actress—finally fulfilling her dreams.

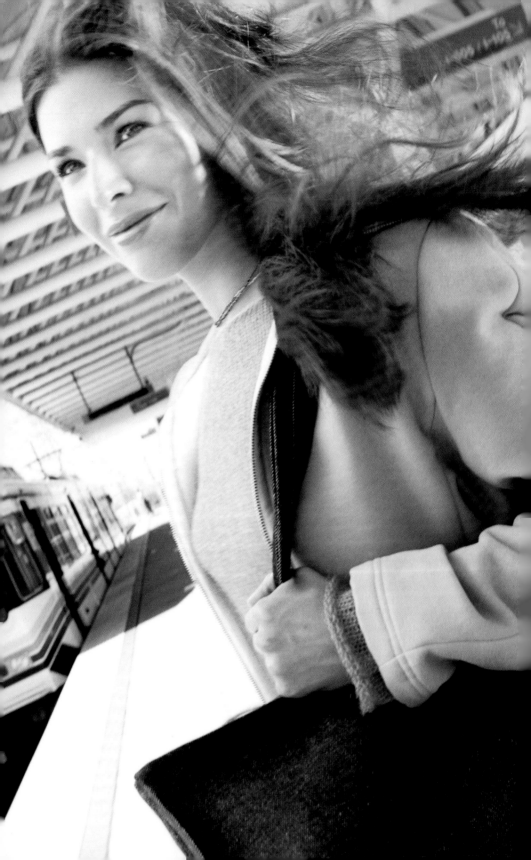

chapter seven
your work

Quick Tip: *If you don't have your dream job, seek meaning and joy by moonlighting. Want to teach tai chi? Get certified and lead a weekend class. Always dreamed about owning an antique shop? Try trading on* **ebay.com.** *What you learn and the connections you make may lead you to making your sideline your profession.*

what you'll learn

Shape's approach to work is that satisfaction with your job and optimum well-being go hand-in-hand. Using this chapter, you'll:

- learn to regulate workplace stress
- discover if you have a bad job—or an attitude that needs adjusting
- banish burnout
- make your job more personally satisfying
- find work that allows you to express your talents and abilities
- evaluate an employer's benefits
- stay healthy at work

how you'll do it

Whether you're self-employed, have a job in a corporation, work for a government agency, or are fully employed as a homemaker and mother, work is truly the center of most people's lives. You spend more waking time working than doing anything else, so it's clearly in your best interest to be content and fulfilled at that job. Furthermore, it's in the best interest of society as a whole to have people working in professions aligned with their talents and interests, since it leads to better productivity and healthier workers.

Yet many experts consider workplace stress to be the number-one health problem for adults, and the trend shows no signs of slowing down. Terms such as *downsizing, lean production, flexible hours, telecommuting, outsourcing, contingent work, globalization,* and *multitasking* hint at the transition the traditional workplace is undergoing. These dramatic changes can wreak havoc on the mental and physical well-being of workers. Studies reveal that three-quarters of workers believe that there's more on-the-job stress than a generation ago.

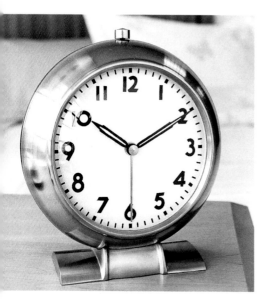

When your job is sending your stress levels soaring, there are both short- and long-term consequences. Initially, your body reacts by unleashing torrents of stress hormones into your bloodstream; and your muscle tension, blood pressure, and heart rate increase. This set of physical symptoms, known as the *fight-or-flight reaction,* won't cause much trouble if stress occurs only occasionally. However, if you're chronically stressed and your body is constantly in red-alert mode, your risk of a variety of diseases and aliments, including headaches, muscle pain, and heart disease, increases.

One of the problems is that we're working longer and longer hours: According to the Department of Labor, one in five Americans works 49 hours per week. The United States also has the lowest number of mandated annual vacation days of any industrialized country—16. Compare that with Sweden's 32, and the 30 stipulated in France and Spain.

could you burn out in a year?

You may have started your job believing that it would be the answer to all your career aspirations, but once the honeymoon's over, what started out as a dream job can begin to feel like a nightmare. Should you be concerned? Answer these questions to find out.

YES NO

___ ___ 1. I hate my job, but I love the high salary.

___ ___ 2. I'm paying dues; I'll reap the rewards later.

___ ___ 3. My job has lots of deadlines and pressures.

___ ___ 4. I believe anything's possible if I just work hard enough.

___ ___ 5. I'm a perfectionist.

___ ___ 6. I routinely come in early and stay late.

___ ___ 7. I don't get much positive feedback from my boss, or help from my colleagues.

___ ___ 8. I spend a lot of my time with workmates complaining about work.

___ ___ 9. I can't remember when I last did something just for fun.

___ ___ 10. I've put family and friends on the back burner.

SCORING

If you answered *yes* to three or more of these questions, you may be a candidate for burnout. When the situation is caused by the job—too much work, too little recognition, unhelpful colleagues—it may be time to think about making a change. If, however, your own work style is the problem, consider spending more of your time on personal relationships, outside interests, and healthy activities. Invest less of yourself in your job so that it doesn't have such an overpowering influence on your emotional and physical well-being.

a new approach to time management

Those long hours aren't necessarily a problem—if you're using them efficiently, are employed in meaningful work, and aren't neglecting other important areas of your life. But for many of us, that's not the case. "The reality is that there is simply never enough time left over to be used for our own health, well-being, or inner growth process," says Stephen Rechtschaffen, M.D., author of *Time Shifting: Creating More Time to Enjoy Your Life.* "If we want to be healthy, we need to create time for ourselves."

For many of us, that's easier said than done. The phone is ringing. The fax machine is spitting out pages faster than you can catch them. You've got a dozen e-mails waiting to be answered. The phone is ringing again—wait, is that your cell phone or your desk phone? Meanwhile, you're running late for a lunch appointment, you need to get a birthday card in the mail for your mom, and that project you stayed up late working on last night has to be finished by four o'clock this afternoon or you'll lose the account.

Mistake to Avoid:

Don't dwell on your limits or your fears, says Marsha Sinetar, author of To Build the Life You Want, Create the Work You Love, *and* Do What You Love, The Money Will Follow.

Does this sound like your life? Do you do two or three things at once? Do you often run late? Is your to-do list longer than a child's holiday wish list? If you're busy every minute, you may think you're being efficient, getting as much done as possible so that someday—who knows when?—you'll have time to relax.

Often when we feel overwhelmed at work, we think that the solution is to speed up and do even more. "We think that if only we go faster and do more, then time will somehow magically appear. The problem is, that's not what happens," says Rechtschaffen.

We cut down on "extras" such as exercise, sleep, and seeing family and friends, so we have time to "accomplish" more. While these survival measures are okay if we use them in the short term and only occasionally—to get through a major annual project, for example—it's not a satisfying or productive way to live all the time. Yet that's what many of us are doing, and it's leaving us feeling empty instead of fulfilled.

"The idea is that if you run faster, you'll get what you want and then you'll be happy," says Rechtschaffen. "But I don't see that. I see, for the most part, severely dissatisfied, discontented people in our society."

When work becomes all-consuming, you put relationships with friends and family at risk; your home is no longer a haven, with chores piling up everywhere; and you lose touch with those things that feed your soul. But it doesn't have to be that way. Work can bring joy and meaning to your life, as long as you put it in proper perspective.

Assess whether you can take back some control over your schedule. For example, will forcing yourself to take a lunch break outside of the workplace help you be calmer and more productive in the afternoon? John D. Drake, Ph.D., author of *Downshifting: How to Work Less and Enjoy Life More*, recommends keeping lunchtime personal. Instead of working, get a haircut, run an errand, or meet friends.

Routinely reassess your work habits. Start with small changes. Rechtschaffen recommends slowing down regularly throughout the day. If you're in a heated meeting, excuse yourself for a "bathroom break" during which you can leave the room and find a peaceful place to calm down. Also, instead of cramming more in, be more selective and focus on what you're doing. There is no stress if your attention is focused on the present, says Rechtschaffen. That's *real* time management.

Work your way up to bigger goals. For example, you could set reasonable deadlines that allow you to work at a more comfortable pace. Unrealistic expectations for yourself can mean longer work hours, weaker performance, and more stress. You could also learn to turn down some assignments, suggests Drake. It's hard to refuse new challenges and their rewards, but with less to do, your work may actually be better. So think carefully before you volunteer for extra duties. Finally, set a specific hour beyond which you won't work unless there's a crisis.

lunch break

Whatever else you do during your midday break, be sure to take time to eat a healthy lunch. Most people who eat lunch on the run tend to grab fat- and calorie-laden fast foods. Gobbling your meal also leads to overeating, since your stomach doesn't have time to give your brain the feedback that you're full. In the long term, rushing meals may lead to weight gain and obesity, which in turn may be associated with heart and vascular disease, says Melissa Stöppler, M.D., a stress-management consultant at **About.com**. In the immediate sense, eating too fast can cause gas—from gulping air along with food. If you eat without chewing sufficiently, your digestive and hormonal systems aren't prepared for the food, and the body doesn't absorb nutrients as well.

Even if you only have a ten-minute lunch break, pay attention to what you eat. Put your food on a plate, sit at a table, and don't try to do anything else simultaneously. Ward off the temptation to cram down junk food—a good way to prevent doing so is to keep a supply of healthy food choices in your workplace, such as fruit, yogurt, and whole-grain products.

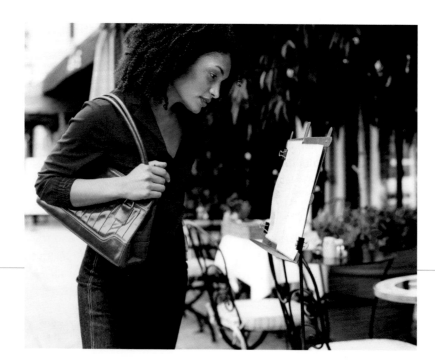

Here are some other techniques for maximizing your time from Odette Pollar, author of *365 Ways to Simplify Your Work Life* and a nationally recognized organization expert who directs Time Management Systems in Oakland, California:

- *Plan your phone time.* Many people find that the telephone is their biggest interrupter. No, you can't turn off the ringer and ignore the calls, but you can be smart about how you take—and make—calls. Don't allow every interruption to take priority. Flip on voice mail for an hour or so at a stretch so you have solid blocks of uninterrupted time. Then listen to your messages, return urgent calls immediately, and save the less important calls for later. Cluster the calls you make into one time of day, and leave detailed messages on voice mail to minimize call-backs. All of the above can apply equally to e-mail, one of modern life's biggest time drains.

Quick Tip: *Realize that no matter how brilliant others may seem, they have struggles, too. Instead of comparing your achievements with others', concentrate on your own successes. List your strengths in a journal, along with any positive feedback you've received from co-workers and supervisors.*

- *Be firm about your quiet time.* You're just about to tackle a big project when a co-worker stops in with a question. You'd like to be helpful, but you're desperate to get this project started. How do you prevent yourself from being disturbed? By telling your co-worker, firmly but politely, that you're busy and would prefer to talk another time. Better yet, shut your door (if you have one) and hang up a sign that says, "I'm concentrating. Please do not disturb." Or if your co-workers agree, set "quiet hours" during which no interruptions are permitted.

when you can't say no

It's great to be helpful to family members and co-workers, but when you accommodate all requests, something has to give, and that something is usually your body. You end up with all the symptoms of stress, deplete your energy reserves, and are left mentally and physically exhausted.

We overextend ourselves because we fear disappointing others and worry that they'll think ill of us. The way out of nonstop people-pleasing is threefold, says Julie Morgenstern, a professional organizer and author of *Time Management from the Inside Out*. First, establish some big-picture goals for yourself in terms of career, family, finances, and community. "Figure out what activities you need to accomplish those goals," says Morgenstern. You may decide that a daily 30-minute walk is essential to your well-being and that you genuinely want to volunteer at the local animal shelter once a week. Once you've outlined the essentials, you'll have an idea of how much time is spoken for. So when someone wants something from you, you'll take the second step: quantify. Morgenstern advises: "That means before getting caught up in the emotion of someone's plea, ask yourself how much time it will take and if it will cut into your schedule." Third, rehearse how to say no firmly, clearly, and politely: "Thank you for thinking of me, but it's not possible right now."

- *Plan on being interrupted.* If it's inevitable that your day will have constant interruptions, then learn to manage them intelligently rather than allowing yourself to be sidetracked by them. Don't necessarily expect to do eight hours' work in an eight-hour day. Instead, schedule six hours for work (or whatever is realistic), and block off two hours for interruptions.

- *Learn to say no.* You're 20 minutes late for dinner with friends when a mini-crisis comes up at work. Do you stay and put out the fire, or let it smolder until tomorrow? If it's a true emergency, you may need to stay, but if it's not, stand firm: You already have plans, and someone else will have to deal with it.

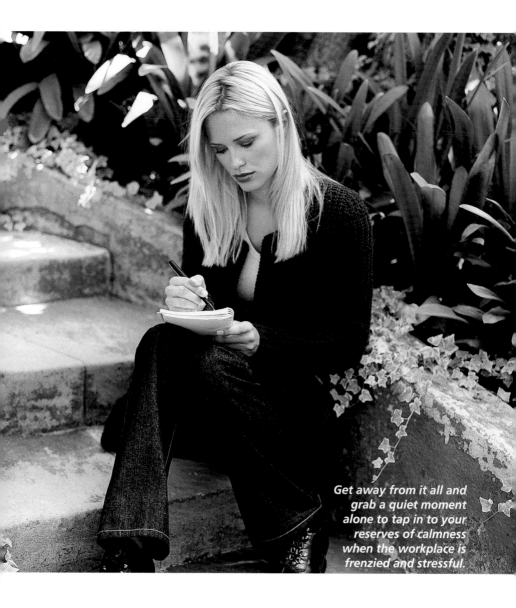

Get away from it all and grab a quiet moment alone to tap in to your reserves of calmness when the workplace is frenzied and stressful.

Be an island of calm in an ocean of chaos. It can be tough to slow down when you work for a company with a frenetically paced environment, but it's possible. Every hour or two, take a few minutes to meditate briefly, do a yoga pose at your desk, breathe deeply while staring at a photograph of a sunset from your last vacation, read a poem, or do anything else that clears out stress and connects your mind and body.

fit for work

Maintaining a fit body can be one of your best bets when it comes to coping with workplace pressures. Exercising regularly will not only give you more energy to get through the day, it can help you think better. Research reveals that aerobic activity might be as healthy for the mind as it is for the body. One such study conducted at Duke University Medical Center on people who spent 30 minutes either riding a stationary bicycle, walk-

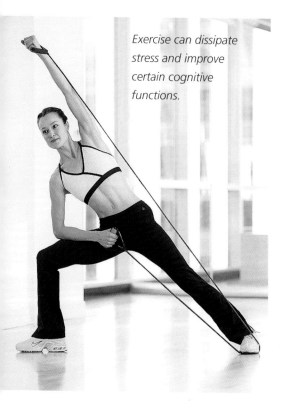

Exercise can dissipate stress and improve certain cognitive functions.

ing, or jogging three times a week, found significant improvements in the higher mental processes of memory and the so-called executive functions: planning, organization, and the ability to mentally juggle different intellectual tasks at the same time. "Exercise had its beneficial effect in specific areas of cognitive function that are rooted in the frontal and prefrontal regions of the brain," says James Blumenthal, Ph.D., the study's principal investigator.

But when you're already in a time crunch, sometimes it's the very thing you need the most that falls by the wayside. One way to improve your chances of exercising regularly is to get together with co-work-

ers and form your own workout support group. Banding together will expose all of you to new activities, keep you focused, push you harder to succeed, and enable you to feed off the energy of the pack when you're lagging.

So find some people who are similarly motivated, and follow our four-week plan to get your group started:

Week One:

Do your homework so you have a plan to offer to the prospective group. Make some calls and find out how much it would cost to split the fees of a personal trainer. Visit local health clubs and request a discounted group rate. You could also approach the human resources department of your company and point out how fit, healthy employees can improve morale and productivity, and see if they will subsidize gym memberships, or, at the very least, pay for the group trainer fees. If all else fails, scout out local parks where you could meet to walk or run.

Week Two:

Spend the week talking to colleagues and choose the right partners. Don't push someone into a training commitment if they're not psyched to do it. And if your aim is to train for a race, don't invite someone in who wants to dance: she will only feel alienated. Pick people with whom you can have fun and who share similar goals.

Week Three:

Before you start your workouts, have a meeting to put your hopes and fears on the table. Engage in a heart-to-heart to share what each of you wants from the training, and what your feelings are about your body. It's important for everybody to feel comfortable with their workout partners. Find your common, core goals. To lose weight? To finish a race? To reduce stress?

Also, set your schedule of where, when, and how often you'll get together. Each of you should write it into your calendars. You might even consider giving your group a name.

Week Four:

Start working out! Recognize that it may take a few sessions for you to find your groove. Use the group energy to push yourselves. Each of you should start to fill in a training log, noting the number of reps, sets, and miles you do and how you feel physically: More daily energy? Better moods? Less stressed? As time goes by, you can look back and appreciate your progress.

the mindful approach

Another highly effective tool for reducing stress and focusing better at work is to approach your job mindfully. The Stress Reduction Clinic at the University of Massachusetts Medical School in Worcester conducts a wide variety of programs and retreats tailored to corporate needs for teaching employees the art of focused awareness. They report that participants in these programs display changes in physical and mental behaviors and attitudes that directly lead to positive changes in work performance. These include consciously responding to situations rather than simply reacting, bringing greater concentration to their work, and monitoring stress levels and taking effective steps to address it.

Saki F. Santorelli, Ed.D., director of the clinic's Center for Mindfulness and author of *Heal Thy Self,* has made a list of 21 Ways to Reduce Stress During the Workday. Among them are:

- While driving to work, become aware of body tension—hands wrapped tightly around the steering wheel, shoulders raised, stomach tight—and consciously release and dissolve that tension. (The same can apply if you commute by public transportation. In this case, your hands might be gripping your briefcase or a hanging strap.)

- Take a moment to orient yourself to your workday once you park your car. Use the walk across the parking lot to step into your working life. (And reverse that process to orient yourself to your home life when you return in the evening.)

- Use the everyday cues in your environment—the phone ringing, for example—as reminders to "center" yourself.

- Choose to have one or two lunches per week in silence. Use this as a time to eat slowly and be with yourself.

- At the end of your workday, go over the day's activities, acknowledging and congratulating yourself for what you've accomplished. Make a list for tomorrow—you're done for today.

- When you get home, say hello to each member of your family and take a moment to look into their eyes.

- Change out of work clothes. This simple act can help you make the transition into your next "role."

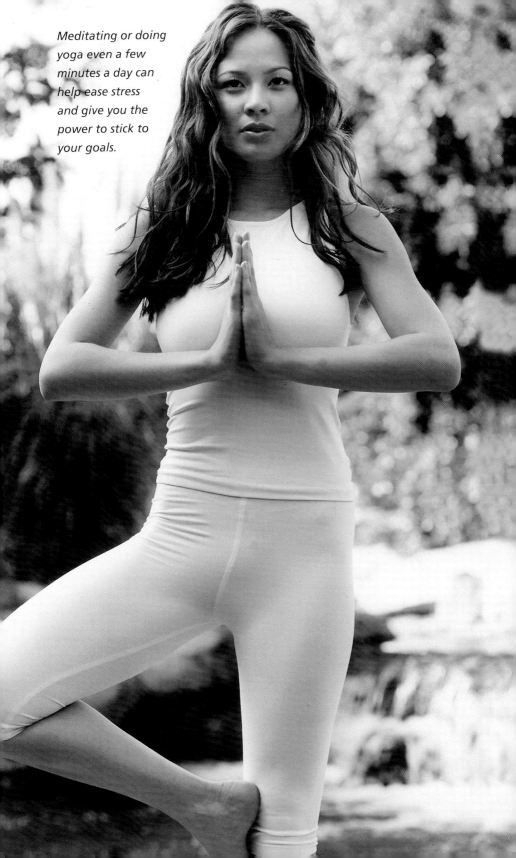

Meditating or doing yoga even a few minutes a day can help ease stress and give you the power to stick to your goals.

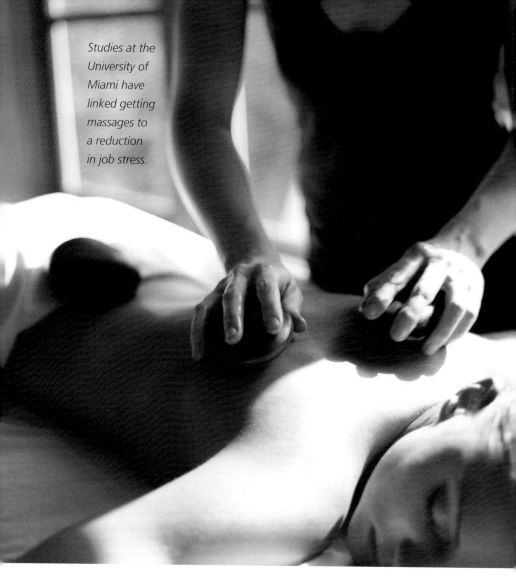

Studies at the University of Miami have linked getting massages to a reduction in job stress.

Meditating is another way to cultivate mindfulness. You can do this on your own, of course (read how in **Chapter 3: Your Spirituality**), but you might also consider approaching your employer about meditating on company time. Enlightened companies are recognizing the benefits not only to workers, but to the company's productivity. In one documented case, the Puritan-Bennett Corporation, which produces medical equipment in Kansas City, started a pilot program that compared 38 people who meditated at work with 38 who did not. At the end of three months, an independent group at the University of Kansas reported that those who meditated said they had more energy, were able to handle stress better, and had few physical complaints.

"Meditation practice begins to cultivate those capacities in us for direct observation or recognition of our own capacity to change, to be more calm or stable in difficult situations," says Santorelli. Those feelings can be a revelation. You might think you're not a calm person, but once you've had a taste of that feeling in meditation, you might start to relate to yourself and others differently. Next time you have a difficult encounter with your boss, you might react differently than you have in the past. "The capacity for non-striving has nothing to do with not accomplishing goals," Santorelli states, "but it's about being more present, more centered."

the burnout blues

What if you feel that all this advice comes too late for you? You're no longer sure what leaving work "on time" means, since you always stay late. You frequently wake up worrying about work. You fell for the earn-it-now, enjoy-it-later philosophy, and you're overwhelmed and at the end of your overachieving rope. In other words, you're suffering from burnout. "Burnout is an emotional and sometimes physical state where you can no longer focus, activities have lost their meaning, and you're just holding on by your fingernails," says Barbara Moses, Ph.D., a career-management consultant and author of *The Good News about Careers*. "Women are more prone to it than men because they think they can do it all. They feel the need to be super career women and set high standards for themselves as mothers, partners, and homeowners as well."

The answer, believe it or not, is to do more. It sounds crazy, but it isn't if it's more of the right stuff. Can you remember the last time you did something just for fun? It's important to make time to do things you like to do, such as horseback riding, restoring antique clocks, or the crossword puzzle in the Sunday paper. "All of us need to do something simply for the fun of it, without any motive of gain, self-enhancement, or reward beyond the pleasure of the activity," says Steven Rechtschaffen, M.D.

"Get a massage," adds Barbara Baily Reinhold, Ed.D., author of *Toxic Work*. "It may seem like a luxury, but it will help you remember you've got a body besides your brain and busily clicking fingers." Some companies even offer in-office massage facilities. Often it's just a ten-minute neck and shoulder rub at your desk, but it can work wonders when you're tense.

Definitely don't compromise when it comes to exercise: It's the body's natural antidote to burnout stress. But there's a lesson most of us have already learned: When we count on getting to the gym or going outdoors when we "have time," we set ourselves up for failure. Schedule exercise as you would any other appointment, and make sure you keep it. "Exercise at lunch," says Reinhold. "A 45-minute workout during office hours may actually increase your productivity."

Often, burnout occurs when you're overworked, but not always. "I've seen people burn out because the nature of their work doesn't engage them," says Moses. "Assess whether you are doing work for which you are fundamentally unsuited."

In *Toxic Work,* Reinhold cites the case of a client named Ellen, who would clutch her upper-respiratory inhaler in her hand as she talked about the differences between her expectations of her job and the reality of it. Ellen's asthma had been bothering her for about six months, ever since she'd realized that her boss had no intention of letting her do the job she believed she'd been hired for. A conscientious employee, Ellen persisted in trying to perform as directed, until her body made the message impossible to ignore.

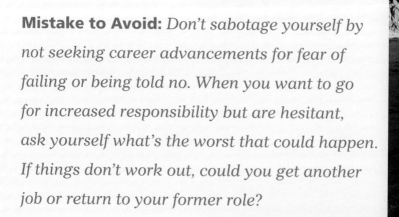

Mistake to Avoid: *Don't sabotage yourself by not seeking career advancements for fear of failing or being told no. When you want to go for increased responsibility but are hesitant, ask yourself what's the worst that could happen. If things don't work out, could you get another job or return to your former role?*

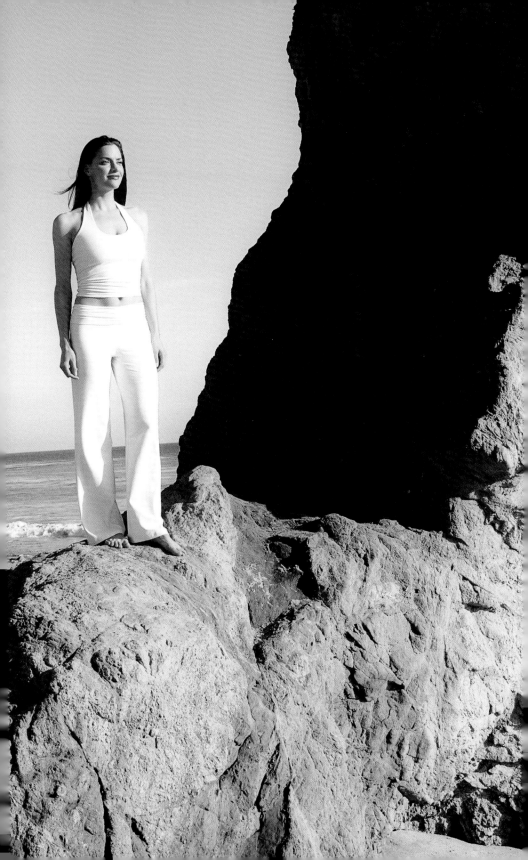

Denying that there's a problem at work can leave you exhausted. According to Reinhold, it's a little like leaving your headlights on all night and expecting the car to start in the morning. Your body will not be fooled indefinitely, and eventually will make sure you get the message.

What Reinhold calls "toxic work situations" present you with important choices that can not only impact your career, but also the degree of emotional and spiritual maturity you attain. "Neither maturity nor wisdom can be purchased except through making hard choices and learning from highly challenging experiences," says Reinhold. Although it might seem difficult at the time, you can learn to use difficult work situations as catalysts for taking control of your own life.

As for Ellen, she solved her problem by spending six months intensively networking, which earned her a position in a nonprofit organization that valued her skills and experience. She took a 15 percent pay cut, but she could breathe again, and that was testament to the fact that she was happier and more fulfilled.

you had a dream

You go to work. You come home. Life is okay, but you really *don't* feel fulfilled. Maybe you once dreamed you'd be doing something else by now. You can't help thinking, *What if . . . ?*

In fact, it's when life is moving along at a routine pace that regret—for not having pursued a different line of work, for losing touch with a childhood aspiration—sneaks up on us. "Many people start feeling regret not when things are going very badly in their lives, but when they're stuck in a rut," says Maryann Troiani, Ph.D., co-author of *Spontaneous Optimism*. "They may be content, but feel they're missing some extra energy."

If pursuing a dormant dream can make us happier, why don't we do it? "Many people are afraid of burning the candle at both ends, but so many people don't bother to ever light the candle," says Troiani. "People become scared of change, or the many things going on in their lives distract them."

According to author Marsha Sinetar, when we become depleted by the daily drudgery of a job that robs our spirit, we can find it difficult to muster up the energy we need to reach our goals. The creative process makes demands on us, she says. It can trigger anxiety, conflict, chronic fatigue, and even intense *resistance* (what she calls the Big R)—recoil, or withdrawal of energy from obligations. When apathy or restlessness undercut our plans, the Big R is usually lurking close by.

Of course, if you want to give up your safe, corporate job to pursue life as a stand-up comedienne, you've got good reason to be anxious: Pursuing a dream involves risk. But the perception that following your heart is a sure route to a life of poverty is largely a myth. In fact, in her line of work, Troiani, who coaches people pursuing a new track in life, sees evidence pointing to the exact opposite: "People who are willing to pursue a dream tend to be much more productive; their attitudes are much more optimistic; and they have better health, better career success, and more prosperity."

Mistake to Avoid: *Don't advertise your fears. If your boss gives you a project that seems daunting, resist sharing your self-doubts. "The first impression we give someone about an assignment can color that person's perspective," says Susan Bixler, a corporate image consultant in Atlanta.*

So, where do you begin? Start with small, gradual moves instead of a major overhaul. For instance, if you've mulled over going back to school for an advanced degree but aren't ready to make a full commitment, sign up for just one class next semester.

You won't make much progress in following your dream until you put fear behind you. We tend to associate change with a lot of pressure and stress, and that makes us anxious. Look at it from a different angle: Examine how a change can really benefit you. Will it boost your self-esteem?

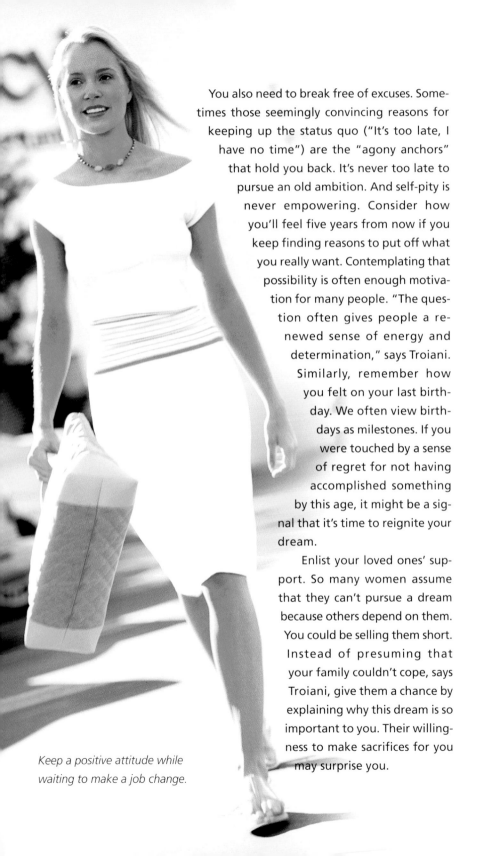

You also need to break free of excuses. Sometimes those seemingly convincing reasons for keeping up the status quo ("It's too late, I have no time") are the "agony anchors" that hold you back. It's never too late to pursue an old ambition. And self-pity is never empowering. Consider how you'll feel five years from now if you keep finding reasons to put off what you really want. Contemplating that possibility is often enough motivation for many people. "The question often gives people a renewed sense of energy and determination," says Troiani. Similarly, remember how you felt on your last birthday. We often view birthdays as milestones. If you were touched by a sense of regret for not having accomplished something by this age, it might be a signal that it's time to reignite your dream.

Enlist your loved ones' support. So many women assume that they can't pursue a dream because others depend on them. You could be selling them short. Instead of presuming that your family couldn't cope, says Troiani, give them a chance by explaining why this dream is so important to you. Their willingness to make sacrifices for you may surprise you.

Keep a positive attitude while waiting to make a job change.

can't quit yet?

Even after you've made the decision to switch jobs or careers, the timing might not be quite right. The industry in which you want to work might be in a downturn and not hiring, or your personal economic circumstances might not permit you to take a necessary cut in pay. While you're waiting for the right circumstances to make a move, keeping up your enthusiasm in your current position can be tough, says career consultant Marci Taub, co-author of *Work Smart*. Instead of thinking of your job as a source of misery, consider it a stepping-stone to what you want. "Determine how relationship- and skill-building, on and off the job, will get you there, so

Quick Tip: *Shake hands like a man. A firm grip could be just what you need in the workplace, according to University of Alabama research. In experiments there, women with firm handshakes gave a better first impression and turned out to be more outgoing and less shy than those whose grips were limp.*

when the time is right, you can move quickly," she advises. It can take a while, maybe up to a year, before you find your ideal situation. Until you can make the leap, find ways to make your current job more bearable, and become more marketable for your dream job.

Refocus your responsibilities. You may be so miserable with your tasks that you're missing out on more interesting ones that could further your aspirations. Ask for opportunities that make you more marketable for your desired job. As long as you perform well and project a good attitude, your boss will likely accommodate you.

By all means avoid the "disgruntled employee" syndrome, where negativity and low productivity reign. You may damage your reputation and undermine your momentum just when you need all the energy and positive vibes you can muster to fuel a career change or improvement. Put on a happy face. "You might have to fake it a little bit," says Taub. "But if you're doing good work, you're in much better shape to make progress."

In the meantime, learn everything you can about the field you aspire to work in. Internet job sites such as **monster.com** can be a font of information. Don't look for "hot" fields unless they're a good fit for you, Reinhold advises in **monster.com**'s Executive Zone. "You wouldn't try to squeeze into your skinny cousin's suit, so why try a field because it works for her?" she asks. "People who are trying to help you will come along and do the equivalent of whispering 'plastics' in your ear. Instead of jumping at their suggestions, take time to consider your options. Decide what you really want to do."

Further, advises Reinhold, don't go into a field because your friend is doing well in it. Get thorough information about areas you're considering by networking, reading, and doing on-line research. Having informational interviews with alumni from your college, colleagues, friends, or family members is a fun way to get the scoop on different fields. Check out professional organizations, trade magazines, and newsletters, too.

While you're still in your current job, start systematically networking, advises Taub. First, brainstorm a list of people and resources that can help you make the leap to your dream scenario. Then figure out how many e-mails, phone calls, or lunches you can realistically handle each week. Map out a networking schedule on your calendar, and keep a detailed log indicating whom you contacted, as well as what you communicated.

Don't search at work, though. Right now, you may not care if you get caught using company time or supplies to land another job, but you could net yourself a poor recommendation in the process. And taking advantage of office time and resources appears unprofessional to prospective employers. Use your own supplies—and the hours before and after work—to pursue your dream.

Even if you aren't job hunting, refrain from using your office computer for personal business. Your employer has the right to read your messages, and chances are good it occasionally happens. A recent study from the Privacy Foundation in Denver found that the Internet or e-mail use of more than one-third of American workers is monitored. Your company's information technology department can also tell if you're using your home e-mail account at work, and can access those messages.

10 ways to make work . . . work for you

1. *Learn to delegate.* Ask yourself, "Am I really the only person who can do this?" Chances are, you're not.

2. *Get together with co-workers* for happy hours, parties, birthday celebrations, and other events that provide a break in the work routine.

3. *Become a mentor.* Share your knowledge and skills in order to give someone else a leg up.

4. *Rehearse aloud in front of a mirror* before making a presentation or asking for a raise, or have someone videotape you.

5. *Do your homework before important meetings,* then ask intelligent questions.

6. *Check your office chair and lighting.* Even small adjustments can make for fewer muscle aches, less eye strain, and fatigue.

7. *Dress the part.* When you feel pulled together, you can forget about your looks and concentrate on the job.

8. *Quit apologizing*—"Sorry to bug you . . ."—it diminishes what others think of you.

9. *At home, do two chores at once* to buy yourself an extra hour. Put dinner in the oven and do laundry while it cooks, or make two meals at once and freeze one.

10. *Create a Friday night relaxation ritual.* It will help you decompress and establish boundaries between work and play.

home-office health

Telecommuting is an increasingly common option today for employees of large companies. Plus, there's a huge rise in home-based businesses: According to the Small Business Administration, they represent 52 percent of all U.S. firms. That translates to a lot of people working out of spare bedrooms or converted garages. Your home work area should allow you to perform all necessary duties of your business without unduly disrupting the functioning of the rest of your household. But more important, your home office should be a healthy place to work. Too many at-home workers let makeshift office space impair their energy, safety, and productivity. Here are some tips from the American Industrial Hygiene Association:

- Invest in a five-legged chair with lumbar support, adjustable armrests, and a height-adjustable seat and headrest.

- Rather than plopping your laptop onto your kitchen table, splurge on a real computer desk.

- Place your computer near a natural light source (how many office workers are lucky enough to have windows?), and look up frequently from the monitor to a point in the distance.

- Work in a well-ventilated area.

- Don't overload electrical circuits and extension cords.

fitness fights carpal tunnel syndrome

It may seem unlikely, but aerobic exercise may relieve the pain of carpal tunnel syndrome. When 30 sedentary people with the condition began working out three times a week for an hour—walking, rowing, cycling, or doing aerobic dance—the pain, tightness, and clumsiness in their hands decreased by 33 percent after ten months. The improvement was probably related to "controlling weight and maintaining nerve health," says study leader Peter Nathan, M.D., of the Portland Hand Surgery and Rehabilitative Center in Oregon. Yoga can also help: In a University of Pennsylvania study, doing yoga for eight weeks improved people's grip strength and cut their wrist pain better than wearing splints did.

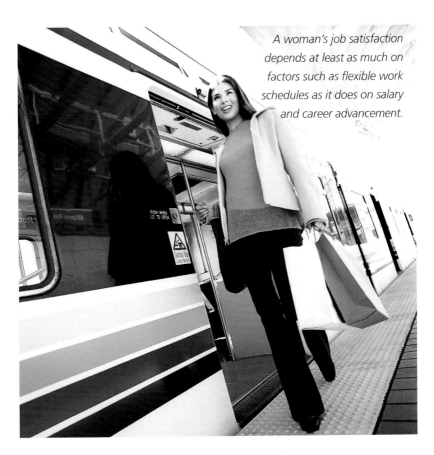

A woman's job satisfaction depends at least as much on factors such as flexible work schedules as it does on salary and career advancement.

women at work

When you do consider moving to another company, you may want to look at whether its policies will be kind to your body, mind, and soul. In other words, is it female-friendly and humanistic?

Accommodating the working woman's juggling act (you know: home and job, family and boss, friends and colleagues, career and life) is becoming an essential business practice. Sheer size brings most large companies under the sway of certain laws, notably the 1993 Family and Medical Leave Act (FMLA), which mandates 12 weeks of annual unpaid leave in the case of illness; the birth or adoption of a child; or to care for a sick spouse, child, or parent. It also guarantees a return to the same job status and salary afterward. But many companies now go beyond minimum requirements. When switching jobs, find out about the following benefits:

- *Compensation structure:* Many top-of-the-line companies supplement a competitive salary with benefits such as company IRAs, 401(k) plans, pensions, profit sharing, financial planning, and stock-purchase discounts.

- *Career development:* Is management and career training part of the corporate culture?

- *Insurance coverage:* What kind of health plans does the company offer? Does the plan cover dental and mental-health services, alternative medicine, infertility treatments, and contraception?

- *Wellness:* The best companies recognize the value of a healthy, happy work force, offering support services ranging from free or subsidized gym memberships to counseling for smoking, stress, substance abuse, weight control, and personal problems such as divorce.

- *Maternity benefits:* Companies with woman-friendly health benefits surpass FMLA mandates by offering adoption assistance, more than 12 weeks of maternity leave, gradual return-to-work schedules, paternity leave, and even lactation stations and visiting-nurse services for new moms.

- *Day care:* Day care for aging parents, as well as for kids, has become the major deal breaker for women. Child- and elder-care benefits come in the form of referrals, subsidies, on-site facilities, or other assistance.

- *Time management:* The most important way of being family friendly is by offering work-schedule flexibility. Many companies now offer comp time, part- or flextime schedules, job sharing, compressed work weeks, and/or telecommuting. To save employees time, many provide concierge services such as ATMs, dry cleaning, copying, flower and convenience stores, and travel agencies.

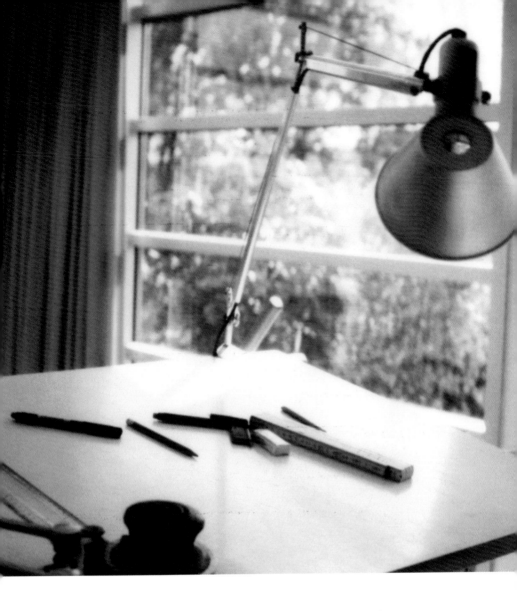

is your office making you sick?

Technology has often been regarded as a means by which we'll carve out more leisure time, but in fact, more of us spend endless hours sitting at a computer. And that offers almost endless possibilities for physical pain. "It's stressful on the spine, back, and neck, and leads to muscle pain and tightness," says Peter Slabaugh, M.D., an orthopedic surgeon in Oakland, California.

"Get up and stand or walk around for a few minutes every 30 to 60 minutes," recommends Slabaugh. When you're seated, make sure your thighs are parallel to the floor—use a footstool if necessary, as downward-slanting thighs put extra stress on your lower back. Your arms and wrists should be parallel to the floor as well as when you're at the keyboard,

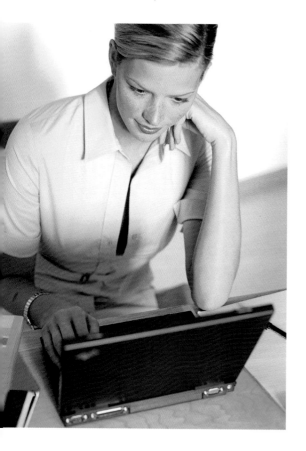

achieved by adjusting chair height. Repetitive stress injuries such as carpal tunnel syndrome, can result from prolonged keyboard and mouse use. Many studies recommend a 10- to 15-minute break each hour. (This needn't be a break from productive activities, just a break from your keyboard.) Stretching and flexing your hands can help, too.

Adjust your monitor screen so the top line of text is just below your eye height. You should look down slightly when viewing the middle of the screen. Your head should be comfortably balanced on your neck so that you don't contract shoulder and neck muscles.

In addition to back and wrist strain, computers can cause computer vision syndrome (CVS). The symptoms commonly attributed to CVS include headaches; blurred vision; slow refocusing; and tired, dry, red, or burning eyes, says Liviu B. Saimovici, M.D., a New York ophthalmologist. He recommends keeping a distance of 20 to 26 inches between you and the monitor. "Large, readable fonts and frequent breaks away from the computer will also help ease strain on the eyes."

the program in action

Gwen Stern was the model '90s career woman. A trial attorney and law teacher at Temple University in Philadelphia, she was also a happily married mother of three. By the time she'd had her third child, she was 50 pounds overweight and fed up with a lack of control in her life.

With a busy career and three young children, Stern craved time for herself, so she set up a bicycle and treadmill in her basement and, to make it more enticing, filled the room with candles. Five days a week at 5:30 A.M., before anyone else was up, she'd go downstairs for an hour. "It was my time to meditate, the only time of the day when I wasn't being pulled in a million directions," she says.

As Stern became more fit, her enthusiasm for exercise grew. She added a weight bench, dumbbells, a Body Bar, and a step to her home gym. Friends looked to her for inspiration, and she discovered she loved motivating others to work out. Within a year, she became a certified fitness trainer, created "Motivate Me!"—a line of exercise audiotapes for the treadmill, bike, and outdoor walking—and was a guest on the television show *The View,* where she discussed her physical transformation.

Stern still teaches law but has given up her practice. "I loved being a trial attorney," she says, "but nothing has been as rewarding as helping others to get fit."

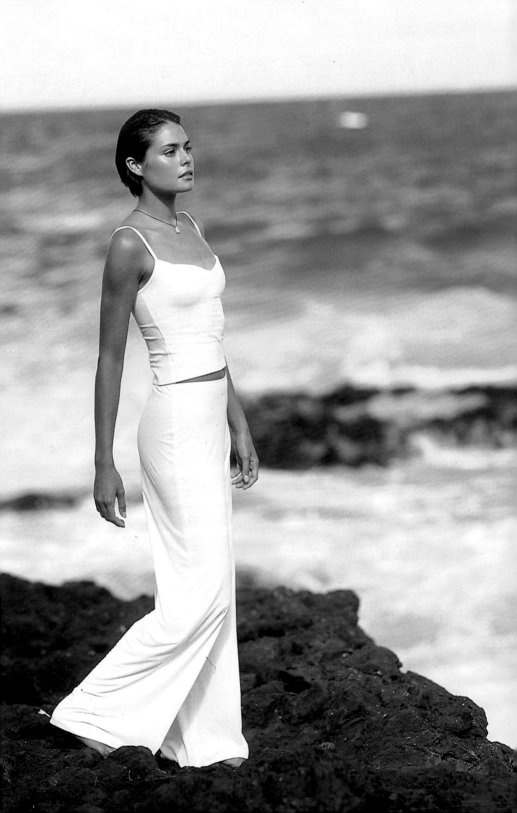

your makeover

Rut Buster: *Explore new ways to socialize and bond with friends over activities that don't revolve around food: a game of racquetball, an afternoon at a paint-your-own-pottery shop, or getting involved in a cause.*

what you'll learn

Shape's approach to being optimally fit today is that it's about enjoying a well-rounded life; appreciating your body and pursuing physical activities you love, both inside and outside the gym; enjoying a healthy diet that makes room for any food in moderation; and tuning in to your emotional and spiritual health. Not having all those elements in balance means that you might need to make some changes in your life. Tuning in to your body, your feelings, and what you really want in life—then acting accordingly—is essential to living a life that feels good, and is good for you. Using the chapters in this book, you will:

- commit to making healthy change
- select a four-week plan designed with your goals in mind
- pledge to be successful in your endeavors

how you'll do it

It can begin with something simple like a pair of too-tight jeans, or a jolt of surprise when the needle on the scale soars into new territory (and you know it's not added muscle). It can also happen with a landmark—a birthday, for example, or the turn of a year—and realizing that you feel unhappy with your life. Then there are those profound life-changing events such as the birth of a baby or the diagnosis of an illness. You come to the realization that you need to make a change, and your life will never be the same.

Deciding to change is easy. Acting on it takes time, sweat, and resolve. "You must move, do, go, and act in order to create real change," says Ellen McGrath, Ph.D., a psychologist and coach who works with people seeking to improve their lifestyle through health and fitness. Change *is* possible. You *can* gain control of your life. But first you must take charge and believe that you can do it.

make it happen

Transformation can be frightening. But remember that it's often said that the only constant in life is change. Just think of all the changes you've already experienced, such as high-school or college graduation, starting or leaving a job, beginning and ending relationships, moving, or becoming a parent. Change is inevitable. So why do we often have such a hard time with it?

It's because change means having to let something go, which disturbs our sense of safety, says Elaine M. Sullivan, M.Ed., L.P.C., a Dallas-based counselor, educator, and board member of the National Wellness Institute. "You have to let go of something before something new has a chance to become," she says.

It's important to be gentle and patient with yourself while you're undergoing a transformation. Take care of your health; keep in contact with people who care about you; read books that provide comfort; and allow yourself plenty of quiet, contemplative time.

"Change is a natural, normal process. You have choices. Realizing this can give you the courage to grow," says Sullivan. Staying in situations—an unhealthy body, an exhausting job, a destructive relationship—that no longer fit is painful and can destroy your physical and mental health.

Sullivan offers these five steps to help you learn from the changes you've already weathered, to seek healthy ways to deal with the stress of change, and to embrace the new change that you are about to embark upon:

1. Look at your life over the past five years. What have been your major transitions? What have you gained as a result? You can even do this in chart form, a column for transitions and a column for the benefits.

2. Are you satisfied with your job, relationships, social life, and physical health? Are you living your dreams? One hint that you may need change is a lack of joy. Consider the potential for positive changes and the strategies that will make them happen. Write them down.

3. Examine the ways you react to change. Do you avoid or mask your emotions by overeating or abusing alcohol or drugs? Make a list of healthy outlets you enjoy—such as exercise, cooking, gardening, or reading—that you can do instead.

4. Focus on one change at a time. When you're ready to make a life change, it's more manageable to target one area at a time. (In other words, don't try to do all four of our makeover plans at once!)

5. Find a confidant, someone who will listen without judgment. If you feel the transition is too much to bear, don't hesitate to pursue short-term counseling.

Once you've acknowledged your emotions by writing them down and talking about them, you'll be able to let go of the past and focus your energy in the present, says Sullivan. You'll become more aware of future possibilities. "New beginnings will come, along with a renewed sense of who you are."

make a contract with yourself

Now that you've decided to change, pledge right now to be your very own success story. How well you do is directly related to the strength of your commitment. Change doesn't happen overnight, but you *can* become one of those women who make other people say "Wow!" Before beginning your chosen makeover, take a few days, or preferably a week, to think about it deeply. Are you ready to make this commitment? Do you believe that change is possible? If your answer is in the affirmative, figure out your mission and how you'll accomplish it. Following is a list of questions, devised with the help of psychologist Ellen McGrath, Ph.D., that will help you get started. This will serve as a promise to yourself that you'll follow through on your quest. Fill it out, sign it, and you'll be on your way to a more healthy life.

1. What are the positive and negative consequences of making this change?

    Positive:

    _____

    Negative:

    _____

2. What are the positive and negative consequences of *not* making this change?

    Positive:

    _____

    Negative:

    _____

3. What are the potential obstacles to my success? How will I deal with each one?

    Obstacle to Success:

    _____

    Action Strategy:

    _____

4. What are my fitness goals? (Be as specific as possible—for example, how many times per week you'd like to exercise and for how many minutes. Rather than focusing on weight loss or visible body results as your goal, focus on process and what you'll do.)

    _____

    _____

    _____

5. What kind of time do I need to achieve these goals? Where is the best place to create it in my schedule?

    _____

    _____

6. What kind of help do I need to do this: emotional encouragement, assistance with housework, or a personal trainer or dietitian for a couple of sessions? If so, where can I get it?

    _____

    _____

7. When I slip up, what will I do? Will I be able to forgive myself, learn from it, and get back on track?

    _____

    _____

Signature: _____ **Date:** _____

Each of the following four makeover plans tackles the issues that *Shape*® readers have told us via surveys and mail are most important to them. The tools for achieving change are all contained in this book—now you just need to follow the custom-designed program that best suits your goals. It might seem that we're giving you a lot to do in four weeks, but many of the programs overlap or converge. For example, several of the four-week programs in our chapters involve journaling. You can, of course, keep one journal for all of these purposes.

tool: here's how to determine how many daily calories you need

1. Multiply your healthy weight by 10 calories for your Resting Metabolic Rate (RMR), the calories required for basic bodily functions. *Example:* You weigh 150 pounds, but 140 is a healthier weight for you. Multiply 10 calories x 140 pounds = 1,400 calories for your RMR.

2. Add half that number to account for normal daily activity. *Example:* Add 700 to 1,400 = 2,100 calories.

3. Add 200 calories per 30 minutes of aerobic exercise. *Example:* You do 30 minutes on the treadmill. Total calorie needs: 2,100 + 200 = 2,300.

4. If you're trying to lose weight, subtract 20%. *Example:* 20% of 2,300 = 460; 2,300 - 460 = 1,840, your daily calorie requirement.

tool: here's how to keep a food log

Study after study has shown that one of the most useful tools you can employ during a weight-loss regimen is to keep a record of what you put in your mouth. Write down everything you eat. The devil is in the details. It's easy to forget about that piece of birthday cake you had at work!

<u>Sample Food Log</u>

*Date:*_____ *Time:*_____

*Food eaten and quantity:*_____

*Why I ate:*_____

*Calories/fat/fiber:*_____

program 1:
your weight-loss
makeover

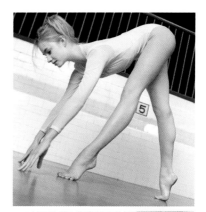

You might approach this makeover assuming that losing weight is a matter of getting your overeating under control, but overeating isn't a character flaw or a sign of weakness. Nor is achieving your healthy weight simply about limiting food intake by self-control. If you're like many of us (and who hasn't succumbed to an entire package of cookies or supersized meal at the fast-food emporium?), you may overeat when you're angry, stressed, depressed, tired, or bored.

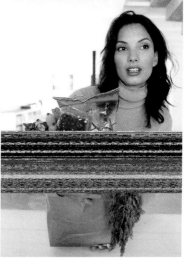

Over the years, researchers have worked diligently to understand the physiology and psychology of weight loss. Based on their findings, scientists now say that a three-pronged approach addressing diet, exercise, and your psyche is key. While you're adjusting the way you eat and move, you also need to get closer to the *real* hungers in your life—other needs that might be repressed through eating. Once you start to satisfy those hungers directly, you're on the road to reaching your optimal weight. That's why all seven elements in this book actually come into play in our weight-loss makeover.

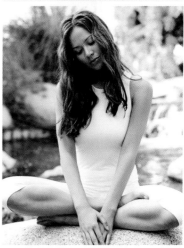

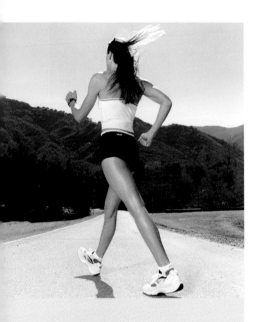

Rut Buster: *Find fresh ways to get in shape by exploring activities that you might not have considered. Figure skating looks graceful but requires tremendous body control and endurance. Synchronized swimming requires strength and flexibility, and the water resistance is great for toning. Orienteering, a competitive sport in which you bike, hike, or run a predetermined route, uses both mind and body power.*

the game plan

What to Read

Chapter 3: Your Spirituality. Read the entire chapter.

Chapter 5: Your Emotions. Read the entire chapter and pay special attention to "Just a Habit," page 234.

Chapter 6: Your Body Image. Reread this whole chapter before you start your weight-loss plan to make sure that you're doing so for the right reasons, with realistic goals in mind.

What to Do

Chapter 1: Your Workout. Do "The Ultra-Efficient Walk-Run Cardio Workout" on page 8 to help you build an aerobic base. Add weight training with "The Fit-in-20 Minutes Workout," page 18. Resistance training is also essential for a revved metabolism. More muscle equals less body fat over time. A pound of muscle requires at least 35 calories a day to function; a pound of fat only needs 1 or 2 calories. When you build muscle, you boost your RMR, so your body burns more calories, even when you sleep.

Chapter 3: Your Spirituality. Review the strength of your connections to people, to nature, and your relaxation or meditation time. Choose a few tips (or create your own) from "10 Ways to Lead a More Spiritual Life," page 145; and take the quiz "Are You Starving Your Soul?" page 133. Begin journaling.

Chapter 2: Your Diet. Do "The *Shape®* Pyramid Meal Plan," page 61. Our daily calorie count is around 2,000. To lose weight, you might need to cut that back slightly. But don't drop below 1,800 calories a day. If you eat less than this, you're generally eating a sub-optimal diet, devoid of essential nutrients that you can't make up for by popping a multivitamin.

Chapter 6: Your Body Image. While you're following the diet and exercise regimens above, also put in motion our "10 Ways to Boost Your Body Image," page 252.

How to Take It to the Next Level

Chapter 1: Your Workout. Intermediate or advanced aerobic exercisers can increase intensity. Read "Picking Up the Aerobic Pace," page 17.

Chapter 7: Your Work. Read "Lunch Break," page 278, and make sure you're eating a healthy lunch every day.

Passion Spark: *Find something you love to do, then do it. If the feel of a golf club in your palm makes you smile and causes your heart to beat a little faster, you're going to do everything you can to make that happen often. The more you do something, the better you'll get at it. And the better you get at it, the more you'll love it. A beautiful cycle has begun.*

How to Get Extra Help If You Need It

Chapter 4: Your Rest. Read "The Sleep/Weight Connection," page 170.

Chapter 4: Your Rest. Occasionally do "The Recess Workout," page 194, to add some variety in your workouts and to feel the joy of movement.

tool: here's how to calculate whether you need to lose weight

The reading on your scale is not as important to achieving and maintaining a healthy weight as some other numbers are.

Body Mass Index (BMI). Calculating BMI, a rough measure that relates body weight to disease risk that's based on height and weight, has become a popular way to determine if you're overweight. You can calculate yours with this simple three-step method:

1. Multiply your weight in pounds by 703. *Example:* You weigh 145. 145 x 703 = 101,935.

2. Divide the answer by your height in inches. *Example:* If you're 5'4", 101,935 ÷ 64 = 1,593.

3. Divide the answer again by your height in inches: 1,593 ÷ 64 = 24.8. This number is your BMI.

The American Institute for Cancer Research encourages a BMI of 18.5–25. A BMI above 25, the organization says, puts you at increased risk for cancer, high blood pressure, and heart disease; below 18.5 is usually associated with a lack of lean body mass and may increase your osteoporosis risk.

But BMIs can be misleading. That's because BMI does not take individual circumstances into account—people who are more muscular than normal or who are thin but unfit. For example, a woman with a "high normal" BMI of 24 or 25 might look healthy but be seriously at risk because she's a sedentary smoker with a family history of heart disease. In her case, body fat is a more accurate barometer of healthy weight.

Body fat. Knowing your percentage of body fat can give you a better measure of fitness than your weight alone. Body fat is what's left after you deduct lean tissue, including bones, skin, muscles, and organs. Body fat is most accurately measured by hydrostatic (underwater) weighing or skin-fold (caliper) measuring by a professional trained in body composition assessment. If you don't want to go to the trouble or expense of getting a body-fat test, you can get a good idea by using the calculator on the Shape Up America! Body Fat Lab site at **shapeup.org/bodylab.**

This measurement can tell you if you have too much fat and/or too little muscle, or if your diet is causing you to lose lean tissue along with fat. A scale will not tell you that. You can also get a rough idea of your progress by tracking your weight and your measurements. If your weight is the same but you've lost three inches in your waist, chances are you're gaining muscle and losing fat.

The American College of Sports Medicine says that 12 to 30 percent body fat can be a healthy range for most women, but 19–22% is optimal. But the fact is, some people will never get below 35% body fat. It's much more important to concentrate on getting fit, since being fit overrides the risks posed by being overweight—up to 35 percent fatness.

Waist/hip ratio. This is a way of determining if your body has too much visceral fat, the risky internal padding around your abdominal organs. Calculate it by dividing your waist measurement by your hip measurement. For example, if you have a 30-inch waist and 40-inch hips, you have a waist/hip ratio of 0.75.

The ideal range is under 0.8. Between 0.8 and 0.85 is borderline, and above 0.85 is dangerous. Abdominal obesity is linked to heart disease and diabetes. There's some debate as to whether waist measurement alone means more than waist-to-hip ratio. To play it safe, experts believe your waist should be smaller than your hips and less than 35 inches in circumference.

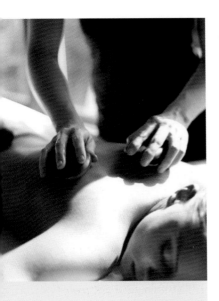

Rut Buster: *Take an adventure vacation: a photo safari, river rafting, mountain trekking, or the like. When you travel, your mind becomes alive and alert. Outside of the familiar, you go into a natural survival mode. You become much more attuned to sensory input because you need to use the information more in new surroundings.*

program 2: your stress-reduction makeover

Does it sometimes seem like your life controls you more than you control it? Continual frustration and high stress levels are signals that something isn't right. It's time to get back into the driver's seat. Reader surveys in *Shape*® magazine reveal that stress is a major concern for many of you, is a big reason for overeating, and that stress-reduction is a primary motivation for exercising.

So how do you keep calm when traffic, an unmanageable child, an overflowing in-box, and a roller-coaster stock market are conspiring to undermine your sanity and your health? Sometimes you simply reframe the situation; other times you substitute smart action for passivity.

the game plan

What to Read

Chapter 3: Your Spirituality. Read "Connectedness," page 137; "Nature," page 146; and "Journaling," page 155. All three of these activities can help you defuse stress.

Chapter 4: Your Rest. Read "Rest: The Pause That Refreshes," page 182.

Chapter 5: Your Emotions. Read "Slow Down," page 211, to learn some techniques that will help you keep stress at bay.

Chapter 7: Your Work. Since stress so often results from work, read this whole chapter, focusing on "A New Approach to Time Management," page 276; and "The Mindful Approach," page 284.

What to Do

Chapter 1: Your Workout. Do "The Mind-Body Workout," page 37.

or

Chapter 3: Your Spirituality. Do "The Mindful Exercise Workout," page 157. Study after study has shown that regular exercise can defuse day-to-day stress. Although pumping and sweating can certainly discharge stress (do those workouts if you prefer; see Chapter One, pages 8 and 18), the slow, controlled movements you'll find in these two workouts can help you tap in to inner reserves of serenity.

Chapter 3: Your Spirituality. Do the four-week plan for "Meditation," page 149. If there's any one magic bullet for helping to become serene, this is it.

Chapter 5: Your Emotions. Do the four-week plan under "Slow Down," page 211, to learn specific techniques to become calm, relaxed, and focused on the moment.

How to Take It to the Next Level

Chapter 4: Your Rest. Plan a vacation. Soon. Read "Vacations," page 185, to learn the many ways in which vacations can benefit your health.

Chapter 5: Your Emotions. Do the four-week plan under "Pursue Your Passions," page 226, to ignite a new interest in your life.

How to Get Extra Help If You Need It

Chapter 2: Your Diet. Do "The *Shape*® Pyramid Meal Plan," page 61, if you're not already eating well. Our diet is not just for losing weight. Eating healthfully can give you the fuel you need to cope with stressful situations, and can help you sleep better. Also, spreading your calories throughout the day can help regulate moods.

Chapter 4: Your Rest. If you have trouble sleeping (a common symptom of stress), follow our four-week plan under "Everything You Need to Know about Insomnia," page 177.

Chapter 4: Your Rest. Take 20 minutes to relive your best vacation, detailed in "Mind Tripping," page 191.

Chapter 6: Your Body Image. If a negative body image is one of your daily stressors, read this chapter to learn how to feel good about your body.

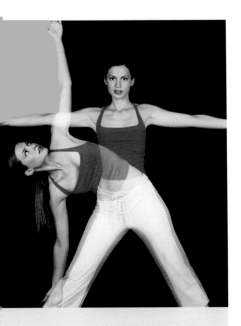

Passion Spark: *Keep your destination in mind and formulate a plan to get there. Having a tangible goal gives meaning to your activities. After all, if you know you've got a mountain biking trip coming up, skipping your Spinning class to watch TV won't seem like such a good idea.*

program 3: your best-body-ever makeover

Have you ever fantasized about running (yes, running!) down a beach in a bikini on your next vacation, actually feeling good about your body? Or perhaps you want to walk into a class reunion and turn everyone's head, or glide down the aisle looking breathtaking. Whatever your personal scenario happens to be, this workout is for you if you have a date in mind when you want to look fabulous.

While it's great to let an upcoming event motivate you to get into shape, it's important to make changes that you can sustain long after the target time has gone by. You don't want to burn out in a fit of over-enthusiasm so that you then lapse back into old habits after the event. In fact, as you become involved in your day-to-day efforts to get in shape, your dream of dazzling everyone at some future date will probably become secondary. Rather than a means to an end, the process will become the event—and you will begin to enjoy healthy living as an end in itself.

Also, in your effort to look your best ever, don't ignore the fact that all aspects of your life—physical and spiritual, personal and professional—

need to have equal weight. When that's the case, there's little you'll feel you can't achieve, and that includes walking into any situation feeling strong, confident, and beautiful.

the game plan

What to Read

Chapter 6: Your Body Image. Before you start designing your ideal body, read this chapter once again to make sure that you're doing so for the right reasons and that your goals are realistic. Pay special attention to "The Message in the Media," page 253.

What to Do

Chapter 1: Your Workout. Do "The Ultra-Efficient Walk-Run Cardio Workout," page 8; "The Body-Confident Workout," page 25; and "The Sexy Side of Stretching," page 43. This three-faceted plan focuses on the essentials of fitness: cardiovascular training, resistance exercise, and flexibility training. Cardio burns the most calories, resistance work increases muscle and changes body shape the fastest, and stretching develops range of motion around your joints, and can boost strength. (In studies, subjects who included stretching in their weight-training routines gained an average of 19 percent more strength than the subjects who simply lifted weights.) When you do all three, the whole is greater than the sum of its parts, and you'll see results faster than ever before. When you work out, tune in to how you feel, as well as the payoffs you receive beyond an improved appearance. Seek to appreciate your body for what it can do.

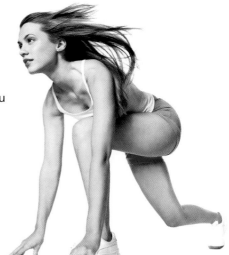

tool: how to figure out your target heart rate

If you find it inexact to use your rate of perceived exertion (RPE, page 10) to estimate the intensity of your workout session, double-check to see if you're working within your target heart range.

Beginners (you've exercised aerobically for less than 3 months) should work at an intensity of 60–75% of your maximum heart rate (MHR). Intermediates (you've exercised aerobically at least 3 times a week for 3 months) should work at an intensity of 65–85% of your MHR. Advanced exercisers (you've exercised 4–5 times a week for at least 6 months) should work at an intensity of 70–90% of MHR. To measure your MHR:

1. Subtract your age from 220. *Example:* 220 - 30 = 190.

2. Multiply that number by the percentage of your target level. *Example:* You're a beginner, so multiply 190 x 60% = 114.

You need to keep your heart rate at a minimum of 114 beats per minute during the active part of your workout. Determine your heart rate by finding your pulse and counting the beats for 10 seconds. Then, multiply by 6 to get your one-minute heart rate. You can also buy a heart-rate monitor to wear on your body, which is a convenient and accurate way to check your heart rate.

Chapter 2: Your Diet. Do "The *Shape*® Pyramid Meal Plan," page 61. Our daily calorie count is around 2,000, but since you're going to be on a heavy workout schedule, you may need more. Get the extra calories mostly from fruits and vegetables, whole grains, legumes, and low-fat dairy products. You can't fuel an exercise program and meet all your nutritional needs on a starvation diet, so be don't be tempted to cut back on calories to obtain quick results.

Chapter 6: Your Body Image. While you're following the diet and exercise regimens above, also put into motion the four-week program under "Exercise Your Option for a Better Body Image," page 261. This will help you to set a goal you've dreamed of meeting, and will give you a longer-term fitness goal than your more immediate one of getting in shape for a particular occasion. Make it your aim to feel more alive in your body.

How to Take It to the Next Level

Chapter 3: Your Spirituality. Read "Nature," page 146; and "Volunteering," page 141, to learn about becoming involved in activities that are activity-based rather than image-based.

Chapter 4: Your Rest. Read "Vacations," page 185, then begin planning an active vacation—one that keeps you attuned to your fitness goals, and perhaps gives you the chance to really enjoy your strong, new body!

How to Get Extra Help If You Need It

Chapter 4: Your Rest. You need to make sure you get adequate sleep and recovery from your workouts. Read this entire chapter to find out how. If you're having problems with insomnia, follow our four-week plan under "Everything You Need to Know about Insomnia," page 177.

Chapter 5: Your Emotions. Occasionally do "The Lean and Serene Workout," page 217 to combine strength and flexibility, and add variety to your routine.

Chapter 7: Your Work. If you find it hard to devote time to exercise, consider getting together a fitness group at work. Read "Fit for Work," page 282, and follow our four-week plan for forming one.

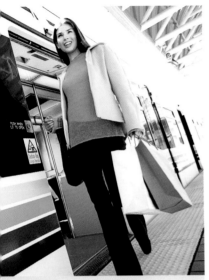

Rut Buster: *If you keep a journal, consider dumping your pen and paper and logging onto the Internet. Blogging, short for "Web logging," is tech talk for on-line diary writing. Check out how it works at* **www.blogger.com** *or* **www.DiaryLand.com.** *You can make your blog available to everyone, share it with certain people, or keep it all to yourself.*

program 4: the live-the-life-you-want makeover

Modern times call for an updated definition of *fitness*. Fitness is shaping your life, not just your body. This makeover is for you if you want more from your life, or if you juggle many roles and strive to achieve your best in a variety of areas. After all, the health of your relationships, career satisfaction, and spiritual development all affect your total well-being. In fact, each of the seven elements of fitness we've discussed in this book affects the others, and any major imbalance in one area can compromise your overall health.

In order to live your best life and achieve the equilibrium that keeps your life in balance, start by clarifying your priorities and values. Once you've done that, you'll be less willing to let competing commitments rob you of the precious little time you have to spare for family and friends, a beloved hobby, or working out. The simple act of identifying your values can lead to better health because you may spot areas where you need to make changes.

So ask yourself:

- What are the three things I value most in life?
- When do I feel most alive?
- Who are the people in my life whom I truly love, and which of their qualities do I admire the most?

Now, circle recurring themes. These are your most important values. Don't settle for second best in any of them. Use our four-week programs to put into action a plan for living your best life. Rebalance and reconstruct various elements as necessary.

the game plan

What to Read

Chapter 3: Your Spirituality. This entire chapter is important to you. Pay special attention to "Journaling," page 155, because it's an especially useful tool for you.

Chapter 5: Your Emotions. Read "Get Intimate," page 221, to get the most out of your relationships with friends and family; and "Steps to Creating the Life You Want," page 203.

Chapter 7: Your Work. Read this entire chapter, paying particular attention to "The Burnout Blues," page 287.

What to Do

Chapter 1: Your Workout. Do "The Mind-Body Workout," page 37.

or

Chapter 5: Your Emotions. Do "The Lean and Serene Workout," page 217. Either will help you feel stronger and give you more energy to tackle every day; and "Create the Life You Want by Writing Your Personal Story," page 203.

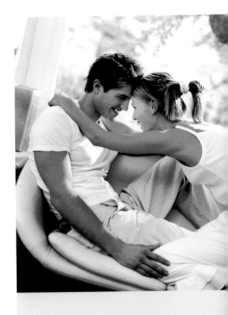

Passion Spark: *In a word: play. Grab every opportunity you can to remember what it was like to be a kid. Do cartwheels. Dive into a pool without worrying about your hair. Slide down a snowy hill on a cardboard "sled."*

Passion Spark:

Need another reason to exercise? Research at the University of Texas at Austin shows that vigorous physical exercise appears to "prime" a woman's body for sexual arousal. In tests, subjects responded more quickly and intensely to sexual stimuli after doing 20 minutes of aerobic activity than when they didn't exercise.

Chapter 2: Your Diet. Do "The *Shape*® Pyramid Meal Plan," page 61, if you're not already eating well. Our diet is not just for losing weight. Eating well is critical to feeling your best, thinking clearly, and having the energy you need.

How to Take It to the Next Level

Chapter 4: Your Rest. When you feel pulled in many directions and overwhelmed by responsibilities, it's even more critical that you take good care of yourself. Read this chapter again to learn the important role rest plays in your health.

Chapter 1: Your Workout. Vary the workout plans to get the necessary cardio, stretching, and strength training in over the course of each week.

How to Get Extra Help If You Need It

Chapter 6: Body Image. Read this chapter again to boost your feelings of self-confidence and self-awareness, and to learn how strengthening your body can strengthen other areas of your life.

Chapter 7: Your Work. Consider changing your job or career, if possible, to become more fulfilled.

And most of all . . . have fun as you
SHAPE YOUR LIFE!

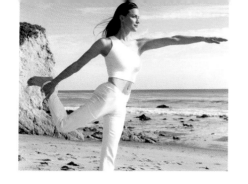

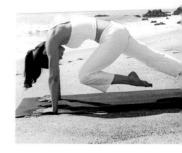

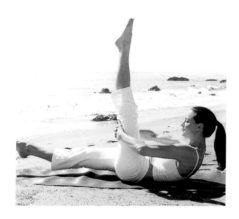

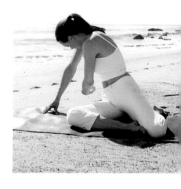

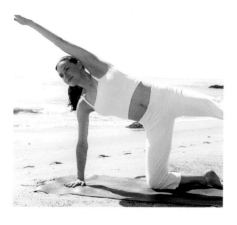

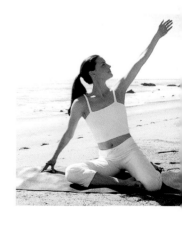

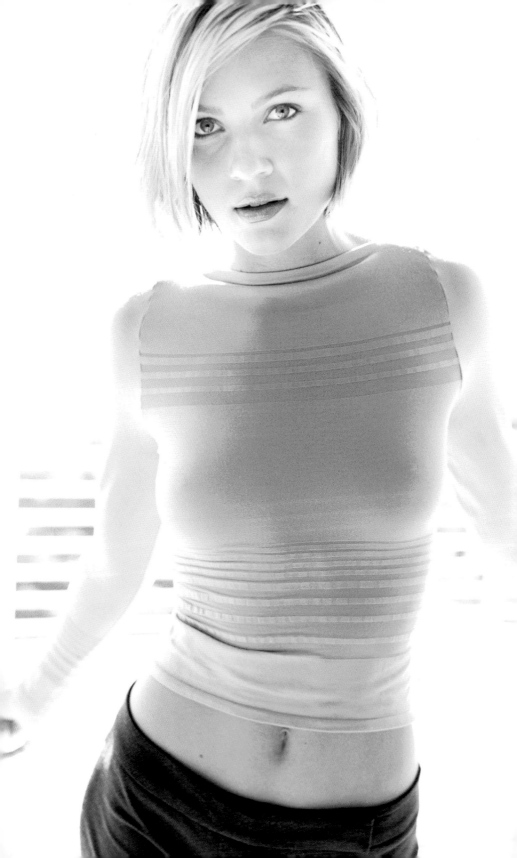

contributors

We'd like to gratefully acknowledge and thank all the writers whose articles, which first appeared in *Shape*® magazine, are now used in this book:

— Mary Rose Almasi, "Trade Self-Doubt for Success," April 2002

— Carolyn C. Armistead, "Soul Support: May 2001; "Spiritual Hunger," November 2001; "6 Steps to Creating a Happier Life by Writing Your Personal Story," April 2002; "Make It Happen," May 2002

— Karen Asp, "Cave in to Chocolate Cravings," May 2000; "Whole Grains: Eat More Live Longer," September 2001; "Home Office Health and Fitness," September 2001

— Karen J. Bannan, "Stop the Plane," September 2001

— Colleen Dunn Bates, "Why You Should Be an Optimist," October 2000

— Audrey D. Brashich, "Fitness Phobia," July 2001

— A. G. Britton, "The Bare Truth," May 2000

— Liz Brody, "Mindful Muscles," December 1998

— Caryne Brown, "Women at Work," November 1999

— Caroline Burke, "Up Your Confidence Quotient," October 2001; "Hate Your Job, But Can't Leave?" February 2002

— Nancy Clark, "Bust the Myths that Keep You Fat," May 2001; "Jump Start Your Weight Loss," May 2001

— Victoria Clayton, "Nobody's Perfect," May 2000

— Stacey Colino, "The No-Diet Diet," March 2000

— Claire Connors, "7 Friends You Should Have," March 2001

— Kathleen Doheny, "Want to Make a Great First Impression?" September 2001

— Mary Duffy, "Strength in Numbers," June 2000

— Samantha Dunn, "Tired of Playing It Safe?" January 2000

— Christina Frank, "11 Ways You Can Beat Stress," August 2000; "Beat Burnout," January 2001; "Is Your Stressful Life Hurting Your Health?" July 2001

— Laura Gilbert, "Is Your Job Making You Sick?" October 2000

— Monica Gullon, "Leave Your Bad Moods Behind," July 2001

— Angela Hynes, "The Power of Meditation," December 1999; "50 Ways to Stress Less and Enjoy the Season More," December 2000; "Plan the Perfect Getaway," May 2001; "50 Ways to Stay Calm, Healthy & Strong in Stressful Times," January 2002; "Stick-with-It Strategies for Fitness Success," January 2002; "Create the Life You Want," March 2002; "Double Your Pleasure, Double Your Fun," May 2002; "Reach Your Goals One Step at a Time," June 2002

— Alice Lesch Kelly, "Write Away," May 2000; "How You Can Fight Fatigue with Fitness," December 2000; "Life in the Slow(er) Lane," January 2000; "Are You Alone or Lonely?" April 2001; "How to Take a Real Vacation," July 2001; "What's the Rush?" August 2001

— Jeanne Kim, "How to be a Happy Black Sheep," June 2001

— Susan M. Kleiner, "Dangerously Dehydrated," September 2001

— Sally Kuzemchak, "Fiber Flap," November 1999

— Richard Laliberte, "Is Stress Making You Ache?" June 2002

— Laura Lane, "Shake Hands Like a Man," December 2000

— Sherri Ziff Lester, "Nature's Way to Relieve Stress," May 2002

— Megan McCafferty, "Your No-Binge Party Plan," December 2000

— Jenna McCarthy, "Go For It," September 1998; "Pretty & Unhappy," "Suit Yourself," May 2000; "Your Body by the Numbers," April 2001

— Gail O'Connor, "Live Your Dreams," September 2000

— Jennifer O'Donnell, "Be Happy," November 2000

— Annie Murphy Paul, "Body of Evidence," March 2000; "Get Happy," June 2000; "Are You Getting Enough . . . ?" February 2001; "Pursue Your Passions," September 2001

— Lauren Picker, "How 5 Women Got Fit," February 2001

— Carol Potera, "Fitness Fights Carpal Tunnel Syndrome," April 2002

— Donna Raskin, "Kick Butt," February 2000; "A Bikini Ready Body by June," April 2000; "The Killer Combo," May 2000; "Get Ballerina Legs," November 2000

— Susanne Schlosberg, "Smart Way to Eat," and Elizabeth Somer for development of the *Shape*® Pyramid, November 1999; "A Bikini Ready Body by June," April 2000; "20 Ways to Boost Your Metabolism, Burn More Fat and Bust Plateaus," September 2001; "The Healthiest Way to Lose Weight," April 2002

— Susan Schulz, "Soul Revivers," December 2000; "The Missing Fitness Link," January 2001

— Linda Shelton, "Power Up Your Yoga," March 2002

- Alexa Joy Sherman, "The Maximize Your Life Makeover," September 2001

- Natasha Sizlo, "Flight Delayed? Make the Most of It and Grab a Work-out," November 2001

- Michelle Stacey, "Sex and Exercise," June 2000; "Starving Your Soul," September 2000; "Your Mother, Your Body," November 2000; "Change Your Body Thoughts," March 2001

- Mary Ellen Strote, "The Crying Game," January 2000; "When Work and Well-Being Collide," November 2001; "The Power of Your Friendships," February 2002; "10 Easy Ways to Boost Your Immunity," March 2002

- Tracy Teare, "Sleek, Strong and Stress-Free," June 2002

- Robin Vitetta-Miller, "How to Read a Food Label," November 2000; "The Good News About Chocolate," November 2000; "Shop Till You Drop (Pounds)," May 2002

- Stacy Whitman, "Fit in 20 Minutes," December 2000; "Top 10 Tips for Staying Motivated," January 2001; "Unleash Your Best Body," March 2001; "The Sexy Side of Stretching," August 2001; "Build Muscle & Burn Calories," November 2001; "The Truth About Fat Loss," November 2001; "30-Day Total Body Makeover," April 2002

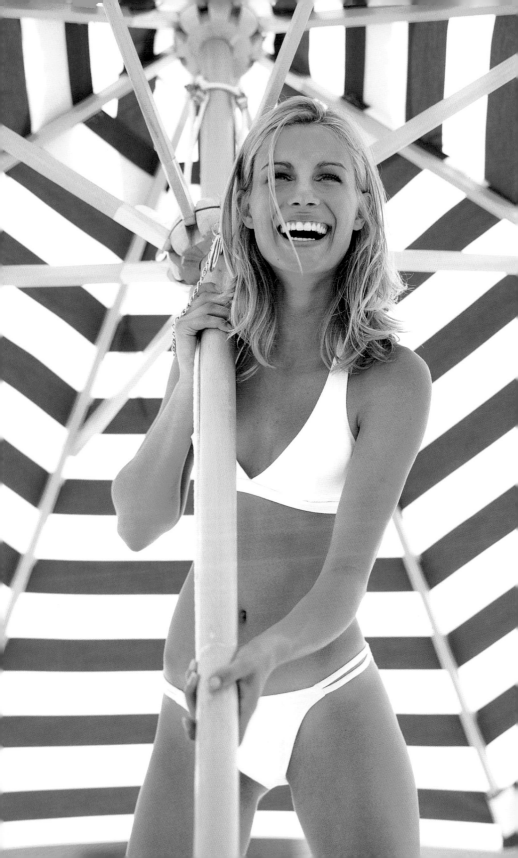

photographer credits

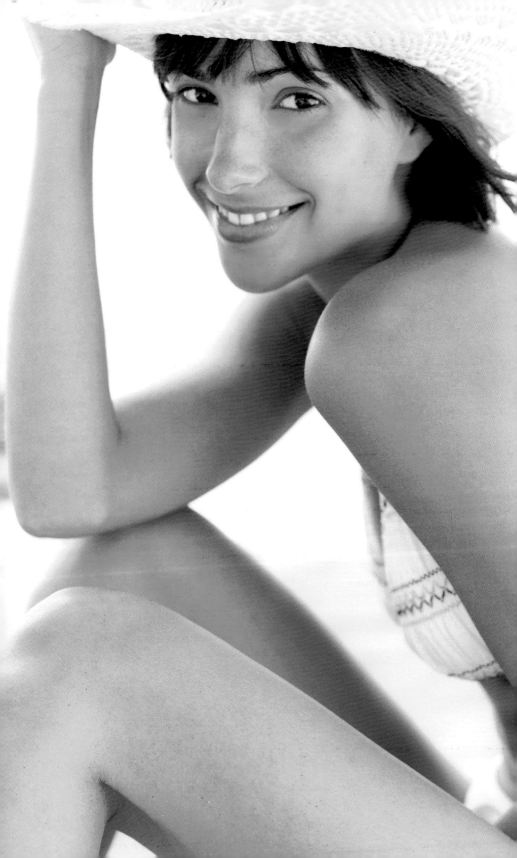

about the authors

Barbara Harris has served as Shape's *editor-in-chief* since 1987. She is a widely recognized expert on health, fitness, and wellness, and has appeared on *Oprah,* the *Today* show, CNN, MSNBC, *Access Hollywood,* and *Entertainment Tonight.* Barbara leads many *Shape®* seminars and adventure-based programs for readers, which are held in the U.S. and internationally. Barbara enjoys hiking, mountaineering, weight training, kayaking, nature photography, and rock climbing—she has reached the summits of Africa's Mount Kilimanjaro, 20,000-foot Hunai Potosi in the Bolivian Andes, and Washington's Mount Rainier.

■　　■　　■

Angela Hynes is a freelance writer and editor specializing in health and fitness. She's a regular contributor to *Shape®,* and her work has also appeared in numerous other national and international publications. A resident of Los Angeles, she practices yoga every day and enjoys hiking in the local hills with her dog. She's also an adventure travel enthusiast.

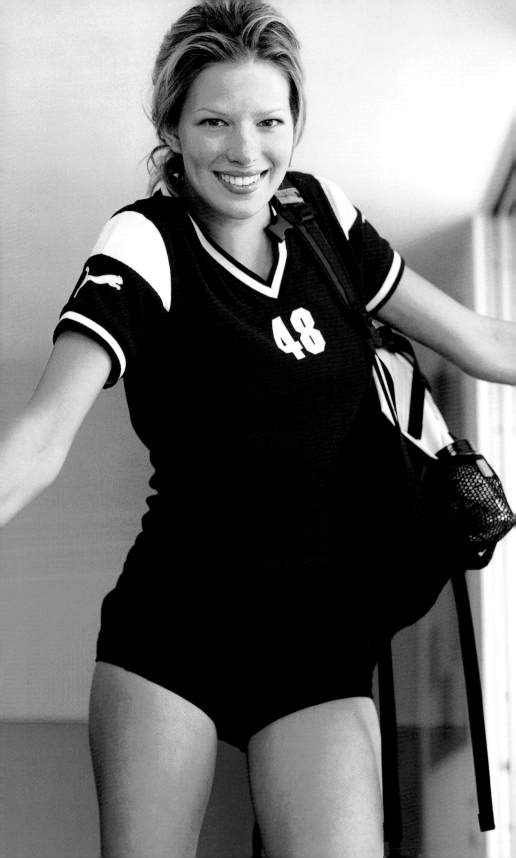

Other Hay House Titles of Related Interest

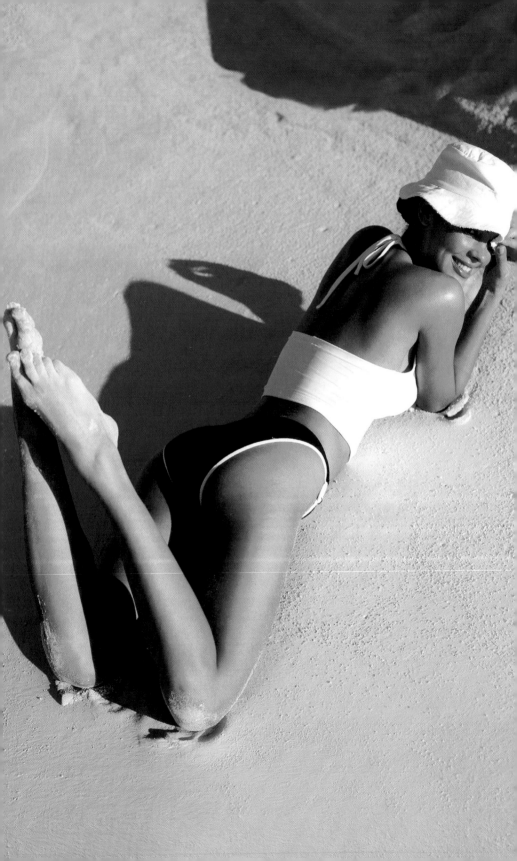

We hope you enjoyed this Hay House Lifestyles book.
If you would like to receive a free catalog featuring additional
Hay House books and products, or if you would like information
about the Hay Foundation, please contact:

Hay House, Inc.
P.O. Box 5100
Carlsbad, CA 92018-5100

(760) 431-7695 or (800) 654-5126
(760) 431-6948 (fax) or (800) 650-5115 (fax)
www.hayhouse.com

■ ■ ■

Published and distributed in Australia by: Hay House Australia Pty Ltd,
P.O. Box 515, Brighton-Le-Sands, NSW 2216 • *phone:* 1800 023 516
e-mail: info@hayhouse.com.au

Distributed in the United Kingdom by:
Airlift, 8 The Arena, Mollison Ave., Enfield, Middlesex,
United Kingdom EN3 7NL

Distributed in Canada by:
Raincoast, 9050 Shaughnessy St., Vancouver, B.C., Canada V6P 6E5

Take your fitness even further.
Subscribe to **SHAPE** today!

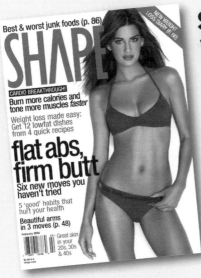

SHAPE magazine shows YOU:

- Smart ways to lose weight faster—and keep it off

- The best moves to sculpt your abs, thighs, and buttocks

- Quick home and gym workouts that get results

- Tasty foods that blast fat and boost energy

You don't want to miss what's new in every issue of **SHAPE!**

- Target training exercise cards

- Pull-out posters

- Success stories

And more!

Start getting SHAPE in your mailbox. Fill out and mail the attached card now—or subscribe at **www.shapeinfo.com**.

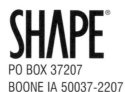
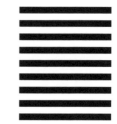